Knickers in the Fridge

Jane Grierson

First published in Great Britain in 2008
by Lulu

www.lulu.com

A CIP catalogue for this book is available from the British Library.

ISBN 978 1 4092 0342 1

For John

Acknowledgements and Thanks

Without John I would never have started this book.
Without Jill, Adrian and Pob, I would not have had
the first spark of an idea.
Without Tim we would have struggled with the publication.
Without Tess, Barbara, Sally and John, my doughty proof readers,
I would have made many mistakes. Any remaining
are solely the fault of the cat walking across my keyboard.
My thanks to all of them.
Except the cat.

I would like to make especial mention, with no thanks at all,
of the numerous publishers who did not have the foresight
to publish this book. And of the two -
Virgin and Constable Robinson -
who said they might and then went AWOL.

1

Knickers in the Fridge

or

De-glooming Dr A's Dreaded Disease

* * * * *

This is not a "How To" book. There are many of those available, extremely good and helpful volumes, written by brilliant and qualified people. This, instead, is my story of our mother, Molly, who, in her early 70's, developed Alzheimer's Disease. This wretched, insidious and degrading affliction slowly but surely robs the sufferer of their mental functions and true personality, and one would not wish it upon one's worst enemy. However, we, Molly's family, have learned to accept it and deal with it over the years, making the most of any tiny positive points and, most of all, learning to laugh. Not *at* Molly, but *with* her and *for* her. We have made this journey with one another's help, and that of dear friends - some of them life-long, some of them encountered along the way, and all of whom care deeply about Molly. This book is dedicated to all who share her life and care about her. It is a thank you to them, a memento to Molly and, I hope, a lifeline in some small way for others who share our plight. If these pages bring you a smile or two, then it will have worked.

JG
April 2008

* * * * *

DRAMATIS PERSONAE

Molly Smith born 26.8.1925

Sally Ellis, Molly's elder daughter
Martin Ellis, Sally's husband
Wenna and Toana, their daughters

Jane Grierson, Molly's younger daughter
John Grierson, Jane's husband
Angus and Hamish, John's younger sons

Royce Smith, Molly's son
Patti Smith, Royce's wife

The late Alan Smith, Molly's husband, d. 1990
The late Nanna Ruby, "Nan", Molly's mother, d. 1994

That will do for now

* * * * *

CHAPTER 1

THE PROLOGUE

4 March 2003

It was neither dark nor stormy the night Mother left home. The March winds had, for once, ceased their battering of the Cornish countryside, and the Atlantic rain clouds had veered off north to drown Wales instead. As though encouraged by this benevolence, a fat moon rose early, beaming over the peninsula. It was just as well.

Whilst nature blessed all with her endowments, the South West Electricity Board observed no such niceties. Although storm force winds and toppling trees would guarantee a hiatus in the power supply to the village, they were not absolutely essential. Sometimes all it took was a whim, a mere nothing, and on a calm night such as this one, you would hear the *clunk* of your electric trip switch as it leapt into the "off" position. Of course, if you were in another room, you would hear nothing, but you could guess what had happened, fumble and curse your way to the torch, and switch the damned thing on again. If, however, you were suffering from the early stages of dementia like our mother Molly was, you would be plunged into the dark without the faintest idea why. With no-one around except the dog, you might just have enough sense left to put on your coat and go next door to Winnie and Albert to ask for help. You would shut the dog indoors, walk down the moonlit garden path, go through the gate and turn left.

Winnie and Albert lived in the house to the right.

To the left was a mile of uninhabited, un-pavemented country lane. Cars would hare along it at anything up to fifty miles an hour. Molly walked on. When she reached the t-junction at the main road, also un-pavemented and with cars doing up to seventy, she could have turned left and reached The Lizard village within another mile, passing the occasional cottage or bungalow. Molly turned right. There was nothing now between her and the Mullion turning over two miles away. No houses, no side roads, no street lights. Just the moon and Molly. And dozens of cars missing her by inches. Not one stopped.

* * * * *

The first inkling that any of us had of Molly's excursion, was when my sister Sally answered the telephone as its strident shriek interrupted her evening's viewing of the TV's usual mind-numbing offers of entertainment. With both eyes, and the half of her mind that was not yet anaesthetised, on the programme, she reached for the phone, wondering, but without much interest, who could be ringing at this late hour.

"Hello?" she said, as one does. "Yes, this is Mrs Ellis. ... *What?*" She sat up straighter in her chair. "PC Who?" She flapped her free hand at her husband Martin, sitting at the other end of the sofa, to grab his attention. "My *mother?* Where? At the police station?" More gesticulations, as Martin looked on in bewilderment. "Oh. Oh, I see. ... Yes, we'll be right there. ... Yes. ... Thank you."

"What the heck's going on?" asked Martin.

"It's mother," replied Sally, "she's been walkabout."

"So where is she?"

"She's at home, Parc Bush. With two policemen. They've just brought her back in the patrol car from the holiday park."

* * * * *

A phone call at 10.00 p.m, with one's mother in the early stages of Alzheimer's Disease, is the sort of thing one dreads. The prospect sits on a back burner in one's mind, simmering gently until the heat is turned up and the saucepan flips its lid. Our mother Molly's lid had been flippy for some time. We knew she was extremely forgetful and that this forgetfulness would sometimes lead to her getting lost, walking off to the shops and coming back the wrong way, or calling on complete strangers for coffee and a bun (or once, more pertinently, a banana). So far, this had not been a real problem, since she lived in a small village, where most people knew about her and would inform us of any sightings made where she had no business to be. A delivery service by the Devon and Cornwall Constabulary, however, was a little more serious.

After a quick 'phone call to get Grandma Betty from round the corner to come and look after her girls asleep upstairs, Sally rushed out to the car, as fast as her still be-slippered feet would allow her, with Martin following, and within minutes they had driven the half mile to Parc Bush, where two constables were enjoying the full benefit of Molly's gratitude. Each was perched awkwardly on a kitchen stool, while Molly, in grade one grump mode, stood at the other end of the room, scowling at them. "What are *they* doing here?" she muttered to Sally as she and Martin walked in. A more enthusiastic welcome came from Tilly, Molly's dog, who leaped upon Sally ecstatically before seizing her arm gently in her mouth.

"They've brought you home, Mother." Sally replied, removing the exuberant hound from her wrist.

"Huh!" was all the answer she got, and Sally turned to the police officers, both of whom looked extremely relieved to see someone other than Molly. "What happened?" she asked.

"Well, Mrs Ellis, your mother seems to have lost her way in the dark, and didn't quite know where she was. The night watchman at the holiday park found her, and called us. She knew her name and the name of the house, but that was all. We had to look her up on the electoral roll, before we could bring her home."

"That's jolly decent of you," proffered Martin. "How did you get in?"

"The door was unlocked, so we just came in. The dog seemed pleased to see us."

"Yes," added PC number two, "almost took my arm off."

"Tch!" contributed Molly from her corner, while Sally relaxed and smiled.

"Yes, our Tilly is a bit enthusiastic in her greetings!" Then, turning to Molly, "So you've been to Mullion then?"

"Where?"

"The holiday park. These nice policemen have just brought you back in their car!"

"*I* don't know," shrugged Molly, scowling more deeply, and she walked off, leaving the assembled company to try and ascertain the facts. Insofar as they could put the pieces together, it seemed that Molly's lights had gone out - literally, on this occasion - and she had indeed stepped outside, very sensibly, to enlist the help of Winnie and Albert next door. Her wrong turnings led her to the lights of the holiday park and fortunately she was sensible enough to walk onto the site, where she encountered the night watchman. He called the police, and Molly got to ride home in state. Not *a* state - that was left for (i) the dog, who was going crazy left all alone for so many hours, and (ii) us, once we heard what had happened and our imaginations went into What-if overdrive. What indeed?

* * * * *

I first heard the Alzheimer alarm bells ring seven years before the above incident, and I can still remember that plummetty feeling in the pit of my stomach. Molly had friends staying with her, and we were all having tea and gossip in Molly's conservatory one afternoon. Someone told a little anecdote and Molly made one of her witty remarks. Another friend added something and Molly repeated her witty remark. We all pretended not to notice, and the conversation moved on, but a voice in my head said, "Oh, Christ!" and I knew that trouble lay ahead.

Someone very naturally asked me, when I told them this, "Why were you so worried?" We all repeat ourselves for a pastime, forget things, lose our keys, can't find the right words, and worry that we have AD (Alzheimer's Disease). Medical experts say all this is quite normal, especially in our busy, stressful lives, and it is nothing to be concerned about. So, why did I think Molly's remark presaged anything different? I cannot say. I just knew.

Molly was an intelligent and sensible woman, and two months later she too realised that her memory was not all that it should be. Her particular worry was that, when driving her car, she often could not remember the stretch of road she had just covered. So, very sensibly, she gave up driving. Admittedly, Molly's decision was made easier by the fact that the car too was losing its memory. In true AD fashion, it would go drive-abouts, forget where it was supposed to be going, and stop. Unlike its human counterparts, however, it would not remember how to start again, not even to wander in a different direction, and it would sit hunched and stubborn by the roadside until rescued by the AA. Molly had dealt with this stoically for some time, and indeed she and a girlfriend thought it hilarious when they were brought home one day in a breakdown truck, Molly sitting in the passenger seat beside the driver and her pal lying full stretch above them in the driver's bunk. However, enough was enough, and the little rust bucket was eventually towed off to the scrap yard to rust in peace. From then on, Molly had to rely on Shank's Pony, the bus, or Sally and Jane's Taxi Service.

During the ensuing year Molly often complained of her failing memory, although, as Sally astutely commented, she could always remember that she was forgetful. Molly blamed the blood pressure tablets that she had been taking for years, so we suggested she see the doctor and have them changed. Of course she forgot, and it wasn't at the forefront of our minds either, so nothing was done about it. She was still able to look after herself, run her home, tend the garden and do her shopping in the village, so there seemed no need for panic.

If I were planning a trip to town, I would phone Molly the evening before and ask if she wanted to go shopping the next day. Her answer was always a carefully considered, "That would be a good idea," as though it were the first time I had ever suggested it. So, early the next morning we would roll into town, and I would leave her to meander while I went off to my part-time secretarial job at the nearby school for two hours. I always left a note in her handbag to remind her where to meet me, but she usually forgot she had this and would wander around the car park until she found our car. It was no good telling her, "I told you to meet me at the supermarket!" because the reply would always be, "Did you? I forgot," so I just counted myself fortunate that she could still remember which car to stop by.

These shopping trips occasioned one of the very few times I got cross with Molly, when I turned up to collect her one morning and found her in her gardening clothes, completely oblivious to the fact that we had arranged a trip. I did not say much, but she could probably see the steam coming out my ears, and she apologised not only then but the next day too. You might wonder, as I did, how she could remember the *missed* appointment for 24 hours, but forget the original plan overnight? Such are the mysteries of AD.

You might also be wondering why I had steam coming out of my ears over such a little thing.   At the time I had not yet met, let alone married, John, my Mr Right, and was treading a rock strewn path through my previous marriage. Add to that financial worries, a new and fairly difficult job, concerns about Molly, and the emissions of aural water vapour are perhaps not such a surprise.

Life was not all bad, though, and my big treat was a weekly session with a Daily Telegraph cryptic crossword. This was a pleasure Molly and I shared, and I would regularly leave her a partly-solved puzzle and collect it, with her contributions, the next time I called. It was one of the biggest shocks I got from the whole AD affair when I picked up one such puzzle a few days after depositing it and found it full of the same blanks as when I had left it.   Molly had solved not one clue. It was suddenly and forcefully drummed home to me that she no longer had the mental ability to work out the answers. This problem, it seemed, was not just a memory thing.

* * * * *

Molly was 71 when the conservatory tea party took place. Her intellect had always been and still was razor sharp, perhaps largely inherited from her father who was a teacher, and her maternal grandmother who had been a governess before she married. Nan (my grandmother and Molly's mother) was no slouch either, holding down a telephonist job in London's West End until she was well into her 60's. Molly had a good education, her primary school days being followed by High School where she gained her matriculation, one of only two girls in the class to do so. "Matric", as it was known, was roughly the equivalent of today's GCSE's, but one had to pass every single exam in order to matriculate. It says much for Molly's quiet determination and brain power that she succeeded, bearing in mind her aversion to history and her shaky knowledge of Latin (the only phrase she ever remembered was *"Tacite, Puellae!"* - Be Quiet, Girls! - which also says much for the school discipline). Her schooling was not the whole story though; her diffident exterior hid a ready wit that could play with words like a composer plays with notes, a wicked - some would say mordant - sense of humour and fun, an insatiable appetite for books and a keenness to learn anything new.

After she left school, Molly went to business college to learn shorthand and typing; such a waste of a brain, being little more than a scribe for some probably less intelligent being, but that was what girls did in those days. When she was old enough to enlist, she joined the Wrens for the last two years of the war, based in Ilfracombe, north

Devon, and worked in the ledger department, which she loved. Her shy smile could not hide for long the bubbly nature underneath, so she made lifelong friends and had the time of her life.

She also met the man of her life, Alan Smith, my father, dubbed (not terribly originally) "Smithy" by her almost immediately and known by that name for the rest of his life. Standing in two queues, side by side, waiting to catch the forces train home from London back to the West Country, the two nineteen year olds got chatting, fell for each other big time, and were married two years later. Smithy's diary on the day recorded, "Married at last, to the woman of my dreams".

Fifty years later, the dream woman was about to enter a nightmare.

CHAPTER 2

THE DIAGNOSIS

Molly was losing things. Her marbles, yes, we knew about that, but all sorts of other oddities were doing untimely disappearing acts too, from keys and clothes to television remote controls and garden spades. Nothing life-threatening, but the more serious side to these losses was that, as far as Molly was concerned, they were no such thing. They were theft.

"Some swine has stolen my trenching shovel!" she reported to me one day. "I know I left it in the shed, and now it's gone."

Because this was one of the first such occurrences, I treated it at face value, and, after a thorough search of shed and garden, concluded that she was right. How horrible. Who could have committed such a dastardly deed? A trenching shovel was an unusual and fairly expensive object, very useful if you wanted to dig ... well, trenches, and it wasn't very nice to imagine some passer-by happily helping themselves and now merrily digging their own pits. Serve 'em right if they fell in. Wait a minute though ...

"You had two trenching shovels, didn't you?" I asked. "Why not just use the other one for now."

"I did have two," Molly sternly corrected me. "They've taken them both."

Hmmm.

I reserved judgement. Then, a week later, when "they" were accused of stealing the dog's choke chain, I began to think her suspicions might be misplaced. Within minutes I found the chain in the study, where it was acting as a not very fetching tie-back on the curtains.

"Here it is!" I said gaily, omitting any reference to her wrongful accusations, in the interests of peace and harmony.

"Oh good," was all her response, and I let the subject drop until the next "theft" a few days later. Molly couldn't find a hat, and was about to start fulminating, so I forestalled her, with, "Oh no! We've been burgled! Call the police!" which stopped her midstream and she just giggled.

She was, of course, just forgetting where she had put things (both spades were located months later in the wood shed in the paddock), and this we accepted as absent-mindedness. We did not even try to put a more specific name to it, and if anyone had mentioned dementia we would have sent them off with a flea in their ear. Our word-phobia was strange, when you think about it. The word "dementia" comes from the Latin *"de"* out of, and *"mens"* mind. So absent-minded really means the same thing; the mind is not where it should be. But whereas it is socially acceptable, even rather endearing, to be absent-minded, dementia is a dirty word.

At this time, we all still thought the actual cause of Molly's forgetfulness was her blood pressure tablets. She had been taking these for years, and had changed the formulation at least once before. Perhaps, if she remembered to take herself off to the doctor, he would change them for her once again, to a brand less likely to have a detrimental effect, and everything would be fine. Even Molly's mild paranoia with the "burglaries" did not worry us too much. She had always been a - let's be kind - feisty individual, and it did not seem out of character for her to make these accusations.

Nor did it worry us at first when she went for long walks and forgot where she'd been.

"I walked all the way to ... somewhere, yesterday," she reported proudly to me one day when we were sitting having coffee, "only I can't remember the name of it."

"Well, what did you do?" I asked.

"I sat there."

"And then what?"

"Can't remember."

And that was the end of that conversation, plus several similar. Then one day, after my "What did you do?" her reply was, "I went to the dentist."

"The dentist? That's four miles away! You *couldn't* have walked there. And if you could, you shouldn't have. Why didn't you ask me for a lift?"

"Oh well..." I could see that she recognised my consternation and sought to assuage it. She hit on the solution. "I changed my mind and went ... the other way."

"To The Lizard?"

"Yes."

Oh good. That was only three and a half miles!

"So what time did you get back?"

"Don't remember."

* * * * *

Molly was an independent soul, perfectly capable of looking after herself, and now that she had no car, and because bus rides sometimes made her feel sick, it made sense - to her anyway - to walk, even on the busy main road. But she would insist on taking her dog (Tilly's predecessor) the barmy, boundful Bosun, with her. Bosun, a manic mix of bouncy collie and wilful Jack Russell, was a hazard to anyone at the best of times, but taking him on walks to anywhere indicated a positive death wish on Molly's part, especially under these circumstances. What should we do?

Another worry was added when she told me matter-of-factly one day that she had had a fall in the kitchen.

"What sort of fall? No, don't tell me. You can't remember."

"No, I blacked out."

There followed solicitous questions as to whether she had hurt herself, and whether she had gone to the doctor afterwards, but she had done neither, so, again, we left it at that. This blackout actually proved most useful for her, as she blamed her failing memory on it at every opportunity, not seeming to realise that she had been forgetful well before that. Perhaps she had had an even earlier blackout, which we didn't know about, and perhaps that was indeed a contributory cause of her forgetfulness. Then, one September day when we were all lunching at Carmelin, my home at The Lizard, she had another funny turn, and I had to help her into the bedroom to lie down. She had been sitting at the table with her back to the sun, so we thought maybe it was the heat, and after a couple of minutes' rest she was as right as rain.

The problem was shelved, as such things are when one knows no better. If Molly herself did not see the need to go to the doctor, then we accepted her decision and did not quibble. If it sounds as though we were being indifferent, all I can say in our defence is that it was not deliberate. Molly was, as I have said, independent, capable, intelligent and, the biggest factor of all, our mother. We had never been used to telling her what to do, and although our roles had changed from parent/child to good pals, they had not changed enough for us to feel we could dictate to her. Besides, even though my "Oh Christ" moment had alerted me to something being definitely wrong, we had no knowledge or experience of dementia. We had heard of Alzheimer's Disease, and realised that it was pretty dire, but knew so little about it that we could not even have spelled it correctly, let along diagnosed it. When half the world spends its time walking into a room and forgetting why, it did not seem of earth-shattering importance if one's mother did similar things.

My mind was changed by John. Who's John? was the question on many people's lips during this time, so perhaps I should do some in-filling. My previous husband and I, having exhausted ourselves with nine years of fights (mostly verbal; I only hit him once), had finally called it a day about a year before all this, and he had left the building. He and I had always said that if (who were we kidding? it was always *when*) this ever happened, we would have neither the desire nor the energy to form another relationship, and for a while I just enjoyed the freedom of life on my own. As Molly and my ex had not often met, his departure had no effect on her and, sadly, she soon forgot who he was.

Within months, however, out of this clear sky, a meteor called John zoomed in and lit up my life. I must have had an intergalactic sign on my head flashing "Target Woman" because he landed with unerring accuracy right beside me, exploded a huge crater at my feet, and in I fell. He brought enough love and psychic energy to fuel an entire fleet of spacecraft, poured it all on me, and has done so ever since. I had never known anything like it. And as you will be wondering what that has to do with Molly's story, I will tell you. It reminded me of how my father felt about my mother. He worshipped her. He had died when they were both 65, and of course she was devastated as any widow would be. But exactly how much his death had affected our introverted but fun-loving and capable mother was not easy to tell.

John is a very kind and easy going person, so one day, when I suggested taking Molly out to tea, he readily agreed and we set off for Roskilly's Croust House a few miles away. Molly adores cake and coffee, so that part was fine, but the conversation was a real struggle. She and I can jabber away about anything and nothing, even these days when much of what she says is gobbledegook (which says a lot for my conversational talents!), but she was shy with strangers, and trying to get her to chat, whilst protecting John from girl talk, tested my social skills to the utmost. To give you a flavour of her reserve, she never addressed John by his name, even in the early years when she knew who he was. I have suspected since that this was because she was afraid of getting his name wrong, but at the time it just came across as lack of warmth. Despite the best efforts, then, of all three of us, we cut short the get-together as soon as was polite and drove back to Parc Bush.

Once we had seen Molly safely indoors, John and I walked down the drive to the car - as one would; but Molly's drive was different. She had recently built an edifice of breeze blocks and large planks in the middle of it, further evidence of her recent paranoia, to stop the world and his wife from using her entrance in which to turn their cars around. The W&W were not, but *we* had been, and it was now very inconvenient to have to park in the road, and then drive a quarter of a mile to the local petrol station forecourt when we wanted to turn round and come back home. After months of this we had had enough. I stopped as John and I reached the end of the drive and wondered aloud, "Do you think she'd notice if we removed her blockade?"

"You spoke my thoughts," replied John, his hand on the car's boot catch, and without further ado, he opened the boot, we heaved the blocks and planks in and beat a hasty retreat. Once we got home, we dumped the lot in my pony's field, well out of sight. When next we visited Molly, she had indeed noticed that her blockade had gone and was furious, accusing all and sundry of stealing it. I earned my first Oscar in my commiserations with her, and she never did find out that her darling child was the culprit.

Such paranoiac episodes, together with Molly's constant forgettings, did eventually add up to a pretty serious list. John, perhaps because he was more of an outsider, spotted the full seriousness of the problem before Sally and I did, and persuaded us to see the doctor about it.   So we made an appointment on Molly's behalf.   Mindful of Molly's likely reaction, Sally and I said nothing to her about her failing memory, but simply said we needed to get her blood pressure checked, and she accepted this.   We compiled a list of her strange actions and behaviour beforehand, and Sally slipped this to the receptionist as we sat down in the waiting room.   Thus we would avoid having to tell the doctor "She does this/that/whatever ..." in front of Molly and, even more important, having her say, "No, I don't!"

The doctor was kind and gentle with Molly and put her at her ease.   Having read our list beforehand, he asked Molly a few general questions and then set her lots of quizzy ones.   We did not know it then, but this was the standard Mini Mental State Examination - an appellation seemingly open to several interpretations - used by any psychiatric doctor or nurse when testing a patient.   Starting with What's your name?, it went on through such things as Who is the Prime Minister? and Can you please write a sentence? - whereat Molly obliged with something typically waspish, such as "Can I go home now?" - and ended with the most difficult example of mental subtraction, counting backwards from 100 in units of 7: 93, 86, all the way down to ... well, you work it out!   Or make yourself an appointment.

I don't know what the score was - Molly seemed to me to be doing quite well - but it was sufficiently bad for the doctor to confirm that Molly had short term memory loss - possibly Alzheimer's.   *No, not that! Anything but that*, screamed the voice in my head, but I just nodded at the doctor as he went on to say that he would get the local nurse to visit.

Sally and I took Molly home, then went back to Sally's place to discuss tactics.

"Well, that wasn't too bad, was it?" I said.

"No," replied Sally.   "At least the old girl behaved herself and didn't give the doctor a hard time."

"I'm sure we can cope as long as Molly doesn't get too much more absent-minded."

Sally agreed.

How little we knew.

CHAPTER 3

DOCTORS AND NURSES

Life went quiet for a while after our visit to the doctor, and nothing much happened. The district nurse never came; no voluptuous Hattie Jacques figure wended her way to Parc Bush on her bicycle, in pristine blue uniform and starched cap; but as Molly didn't actually need a nurse, this didn't bother us. Molly had, it seemed, settled into a routine. She forgot things, but nothing life-threatening. She went for walks, never remembering where but always finding her way home. She lost garden shears, secateurs and trowels, but who doesn't? When she mislaid the television remote yet again, John found it under the sofa and tied it to her chair. When she couldn't find her back door key, we chained the spare one to the wall by the door. She continued to keep a neat garden and a tidy home. She did her own shopping, walking down to the village shop with her trolley basket, loading it with sausages, cake and Bosun-dog's Winalot and wheeling it home again. As she didn't always think to take house-keeping money out of the Post Office, I made sure there was always some cash in her purse. If I couldn't find the purse immediately, I would leave £5 with a note attached; "shopping money". If she mislaid her handbag, which she did frequently, she would put off her shopping trip until she found it. Sally explained the situation to the local shop-keeper so that there was no risk of Molly being accused of shoplifting or coming home with an empty basket, and they became used to her and to her strange purchases. They were also very helpful with taking the right money from her so that she only needed to hold out a handful of coins on her palm for them to help themselves.

As summer approached, Sally and I each visited Molly a couple of times a week, and I would sometimes bring her over to Carmelin for supper, Bosun at her side as always. I noticed that her appetite had decreased and she was looking thinner, but I couldn't think why. Her larder was, as ever, chock full of cakes and biscuits and it was not as though she was forgetting to eat. It was just possible that the ever expanding Bosun was getting a heck of a lot more carbohydrates than she was, but I also wondered if she might have developed diabetes, so I took her off to the surgery again for a check-up. The doctor, after giving her a thorough examination, put my mind at rest.

"There's nothing much wrong, really," he said. "She has a minor problem with an under-active thyroid, but I can give her some pills that will help. Other than that, all I can say is that weight loss tends to occur in people with your mother's problem." I much appreciated his discreet lack of reference to dementia, but Molly, if she even noticed, said not a word and asked no questions. So we added another packet of pills to Molly's daily intake, hoping that she would remember to take them and that they would prove helpful.

In contrast to her decreasing weight, it seemed that Molly's social life was now developing nicely, and she told me all about it one morning when we were sitting guzzling coffee and cake in her conservatory. Excuse me, but at this point I really must stop calling it a *conservatory*. In our family it is known as a sherb. In 1989, when it was built, Sally's eldest child, Wenna, was but four years old, and when Molly told her she had had a conservatory built, Wenna solemnly repeated this to her mama.

"Molly's got a sherbetcy," she announced.

Like so many childish malapropisms, this one stuck, but became shortened to sherb. John and I have one at Carmelin too. So, there were Molly and I, in her sherb, partaking of a refreshing cuppa, and admiring her pretty and well-tended garden, when she told me, "Two ladies visited me yesterday."

"Oh? Who was that then?"

"I don't know."

Sigh. Here we go. "Well, what did they want?"

"They didn't say. I offered them a cup of tea."

"And did they stay?"

"Well, I think one of them had a drink of water, then they left."

"Really? Perhaps they were walkers doing the coast path and got thirsty."

We agreed on this solution, odd though it seemed. Parc Bush is not on the coast path; in fact it is some distance inland on a fairly busy road, not the sort that anyone would choose to walk along for pleasure. But what was the use of more questions? It would only serve to distress Molly, and our firm policy now was to Keep Mother Happy. We would brush aside any- and everything, in her presence, to stop her from worrying and to make her feel that she was perfectly normal. AD experts we were not, but this seemed the natural thing to do, and was, we learned later, the very best approach we could have adopted.

Molly's mystery visitors were followed a short time later by a mystery phone call.

"Somebody phoned me yesterday," Molly stated, "to ask if I would like to talk to someone about my loss of memory."

"And what did you say?" I asked, expecting the usual "Can't remember", but she surprised me by answering, "I told them No thank you."

"Well, who was it? Do you know?"

"Haven't a clue."

This was too much. I rang the surgery next day and spoke at some length to the doctor, asking what would have been said to Molly and indeed who would have said it. He informed me that it would have been the community psychiatric nurse (CPN), and/or the Occupational Therapist from a clinic in Redruth, about 25 miles away. I had never heard of this clinic. Why would I? But the doctor explained that it was a semi-independent unit for psychiatric patients, part funded by the local council, and that its staff did what they could to help patients like Molly. I was astounded to learn that she had been visited in December, January and May and consequently referred to the consultant service. This explained the mystery visitors; they had been the CPN and OT - not the district nurse at all. It also explained the phone calls, of which there had been three, each one resulting in an out-patient appointment, and each appointment cancelled by Molly, simply because she did not understand what was going on. The clinic had therefore discharged Molly from its care.

I was further amazed that anyone from the medical profession had actually contacted Molly when they were all fully aware of her condition. They had severely overestimated her mental abilities, and even if she had been able to remember the visits and phone calls, how did they expect her to get to Redruth? Or remember to ask anyone for help? However, their hearts were obviously in the right place, so I trod gently. I wrote a lengthy letter to the clinic, requesting that Molly be reinstated on the consultancy referral list, and asked "What now?"

As a family, our difficulty lay in not wishing to take charge of Molly's life when it was not necessary, and in helping her to retain the dignity of independence as far as, and for as long as, possible, whilst at the same time wanting to pursue any avenue which might help her to cope; including the clinic's offer which she had refused. I suggested that the CPN keep in touch with me or Sally, rather than Molly, so that we could approach Molly when we judged the mood was right and gently steer her towards the right decision. In this way, an appointment was made for Molly to see the consultant in September 2000.

At a distance of years, I cannot now remember how much of the truth I told Molly about this impending visit. Being a well brought up daughter, and having as a mother someone who would die rather than lie, it did not come naturally to me to tell porky pies. A sin of omission, however, is a different matter, and as the years have gone by, we have told her less and less, but always with her welfare in mind. At that time, I knew her well enough to realise that she would object to anyone poking and prying into her life, so I might just have said we were going shopping, and then gone on to the surgery for a surprise "blood pressure" visit. I cannot recall. But I do recall the consultant.

After the usual spell in the dreary waiting room, where Molly and I each passed the time with a five year old copy of Knitting Monthly, we were called in to the surgery, to be greeted by the OT, and ... a doctor in a white coat? No, an extremely large lady, wrapped in voluminous, multi-coloured skirts and blouses, and sporting the most serious pair of Doc Martin boots you have ever seen. This was Dr B, our delightful lady consultant, and she greeted us with a chubby, sunny smile.

Introductions made, Dr B took Molly through the Mini Mental State Exam, while I sat willing my mother to get the answers right. So much for my willpower; she found many questions beyond her, but Dr B was not fazed. "I think we can help you with something," she beamed, and took up her pen. Another prescription? A change of blood pressure pills? Neither. Reaching forward on her desk, she pulled towards her a large pad entitled "History Sheet of Hospital/Clinical Notes", and proceeded to draw a masterpiece. I have it to this day. It resembled nothing so much as a large tadpole sprouting a flower from its head, a dog bone hovering over that, and three small spiders dancing a quadrille in the bottom right hand corner. Scribbled here and there were words such as synapse, acetyl choline, seratonin, dopamine and Ma. Only the last made any sense to me - although it seemed odd for the consultant to use so familiar a term in reference to her patient - but the drawings themselves were apparently Molly's brain cells, and the dog bone and sprouting tadpole were not connecting across the synapse as they should, owing to a lack of the acetyl stuff. This was where a prescription could help, because a fairly new drug called Arricept would help to increase the acetyl and thus give the nerves a boost in whizzing their messages across the synapses. For a while anyway. And I never did find out what Ma meant.

Dr B might have told me at this meeting that Arricept was also an anti-depressant, but if she did, it didn't register. We were not aware of Molly being depressed, and besides, at this time the only thing that interested us was addressing the memory problem. The anti-depressant ingredient did actually kick in very shortly, but in the meantime there were yet more benefits to arise, the main one of which was financial. The consultancy service would help us to apply for Attendance Allowance (AA). We had heard of this, because our Nan qualified for it during her last few years, and we had thus gained £3 each for putting her to bed every night. By now the allowance was more substantial, and, what was more, we didn't even have to fill out the form. Liz, the CPN, came to Carmelin and did it for us. She knew exactly what to write in order to ensure that Molly received the benefit.

Liz also said something that registered immediately and deeply in my consciousness. *Sometimes you will think your mother is being deliberately difficult, but she is not – she cannot help forgetting.* This was the best piece of advice she could have given us. Sometimes when it seems impossible to take in the extent to which Molly cannot remember things, I just tell myself that it is like expecting a person with a broken leg to get up and walk. That is it, in a nutshell. And it should be issued as a warning with every diagnosis of Alzheimer's Disease, so that the carer knows a little of what to expect.

Within a few weeks of Liz's visit, we had a letter from the council to say that Molly would receive a weekly AA sum paid into her account. A large cheque for the backdated total was included.

I made the mistake of recounting the whole tale to Molly, telling her to listen carefully, and was she appreciative!

Was she? No, she wasn't.

"How ridiculous!" she expostulated. "What a waste of money! I am quite capable of looking after myself and I don't need any handouts from anyone, thank you very much."

I just repeated silently the last four words of her sentence. I knew how essential the AA would be, and was very thankful indeed.

I had taken over all Molly's accounts a few months before this because she was finding them increasingly hard to deal with. All her books were in immaculate order, so it was easy to know exactly what was happening in her financial world. Not a lot. She could manage, but there was nothing to spare. Sally and I brought our brother Royce in on the situation, and on a combined business and pleasure trip to the inn at Bodinnick, run by Royce and his wife Patti, we reviewed Molly's finances over lunch. Replete and genial after an Old Ferry Inn offering, we sat back and waited for inspiration over the coffee cups.

"Well," said Royce brightly, "if Mother can't manage, perhaps we can have a whip-round and all donate a little something each month?"

A split second of silence was followed by a chorus:

Sally: "Not from me! We're on Family Credit!"

Jane: "I get paid for an eight hour week!"

Royce: "Well, I've got a £12,000 overdraft!"

So that was the end of Royce's bright idea. The AA was essential.

As for the backdated payment, I would approach this subject another way. A few days later, when I called on Molly, I mentioned casually, "I've just got your bank statement, and guess what! You've got about a hundred pounds more than I thought you had!"

Molly was sufficiently disassociated from her finances, and sufficiently trustful of me, to swallow this. "Ooh, have I really? We'll have to have a party!"

So Sally and I arranged one, a meal for everyone at our favourite local restaurant. Sally and Martin, daughters Wenna and Toana, John and I, and John's two boys, Angus and Hamish, who were staying with us that weekend. It was a real family gathering. Except that the star of the show did not appear. Molly stayed at home.

It was so sad. When Sally and Martin called to collect her, Molly was having a leisurely bath before an early bedtime, and was quite unprepared for an evening out. She and Sally had a shouted conversation through the bathroom door, Molly saying she thought the meal had been arranged for the next night, Sally saying no but insisting that she was happy to wait while Molly dressed. Molly, sadly, went into completely negative mode, saying she wasn't prepared, wouldn't be rushed, couldn't be ready inside an hour, was not in the mood, wasn't hungry etc. Sally wisely left it. She never had stood up to Mother and was not about to start now. This was our first encounter with the Sundowner Syndrome, or evening depression, although we did not recognise it at the time, and it was the AD speaking more than Molly. Even the Arricept was not proof against her feeling of not being able to cope. The old Molly would have quietly enjoyed a gathering of the clans, and would have fallen in with any last minute plans. This new Molly could not quite face it.

CHAPTER 4

DOGGEDLY ON

A November evening, and it was supper time at Carmelin. This entailed my throwing several vegetables and garlic cloves into a frying pan, some pasta into a saucepan, and a glass or three of wine down my throat. It was a relaxed, winding-down time, and I was enjoying myself as usual, humming tunelessly, opening and shutting cupboard and fridge doors to see whether this would reveal any hitherto undiscovered ingredient to enhance the menu (usually not), and seeing how long it would take John to come and offer to pour the drinks (he was always too late). He duly appeared, just as I remembered aloud that I should call Molly.

"Why now?" he asked, puzzled. "Are you going to invite her to supper?"

"To eat *this*? No, I want to see if the vet came this afternoon."

I had been with Molly a few hours before, and was distressed to see Bosun not at all well. Molly had adored her dog for the last 11 years, but due to Molly's feeding and disciplinary regimes, this hairy but lovable mutt was a huge and uncontrollable lump of a dog. He would aim his considerable bulk enthusiastically at any one of us when we visited, leaping as high as he was able and rushing around in joyful circles, but today he had been lying on the floor under the table and able to manage but one feeble thump of his tail on the carpet.

"What's wrong with him?" I had asked Molly worriedly.

"Don't know. I talked to the vet, but he didn't know either."

I was not sure how much accuracy I could attach to this statement, so I got on the phone to the surgery immediately and said that the dog seemed to be on the point of collapse. Indeed, in view of his prostrate position, he seemed to have reached that point already. The receptionist said that the vet was out on the road at the moment but would call as soon as possible. He had visited Bosun at Parc Bush before, knew the way and knew the dog, so I left it at that. Molly did not seem unduly worried.

I came home, and forgot about the problem until the evening. I stopped cooking for a moment, and rang Molly. "Just wondered what the vet said about Bosun," I said, expecting ... I don't know ... the usual tale of pills and antibiotic injections. Molly was silent for a split second and I thought, She's forgotten. Then she said, "Bosun is dead."

"Oh, Mother, no!" I cried, "When?"

"He died before the vet got here."

I could not say another word. "I'll ring you back," I managed to splutter, and burst into tears. Poor, dear boy. Eleven years was not a great age for a mongrel, and although he had been overweight, unhealthy and lumpy, I never dreamed he was so ill. It was a horrible shock.

Molly too was distraught. Besides being a dog lover all her life, showering the family mongrels with more love and attention than she gave us, her children, she had been particularly close to Bosun. He had been her pal, especially since Smithy died ten years before - ironically, to the day. The whole thing was too horrible for words. Martin was prepared to go and bury the old fellow in the garden, but Molly did it herself that very night and, not being able to dig very deep, on account of the lost trenching shovel, did not do a very good job of it. A few days later, the fox discovered the spot and did some digging of his own. He gave up fairly soon, but disturbed enough earth to leave a hairy Bosun paw uncovered, which of course distressed Molly even more.

After the tears, Molly's reaction to the tragedy was sensible enough. She wanted another dog immediately. Not a puppy but something more mature, preferably small, that needed a home, so she set about phoning vets, RSPCA, rescue centres and local kennels; all to no avail. We could hardly believe that there did not seem to be one homeless hound on the Lizard Peninsula. Sally and I advocated patience to Molly, but she wasn't having any of it. She wanted a dog and she wanted it NOW. I happened to mention this to Liz, our CPN, just in passing, and was surprised when Liz said to try and dissuade Molly from having a dog at all. I didn't understand why, and I guess I didn't ask, because I cannot recall any reason being given. Something like "She will forget to feed it," might have been helpful, but still I doubt that any of us would have taken notice. We are such a doggy family, and Sally and I would happily have attended to the feeding ourselves if necessary. Besides, we knew that a dog would be essential company for Molly. And besides again, there was no gainsaying Mother. So I began my own search.

The Helston Free Gazette answered our prayers. Two collies and a Staffie cross were presently residing, awaiting good homes, at Lands End Kennels. A long way away, but those were the only three dogs available until after Christmas when the usual sad sackfuls of unwanted Christmas present puppies would be dumped there. So, on 16 December, John, Molly and I set off on Mission Mutt. The collies were huge. They would need lots of exercise, and I knew full well that Molly did not do taking dogs for walks. So, onto the next pen, with the slightly smaller Staffie cross, a six month old bitch called Tilly. Tilly went into orbit when the kennel maid appeared, jumping all over her in ecstasy, and taking hold of her arm very gently in her mouth. How sweet and lovable, we thought. The girl put Tilly on a lead, invited Molly to walk her round the field, which we all did, and Tilly behaved like a real lady. While we were walking this perfect specimen, I whispered to Molly, "If they ask, tell them you'll walk the dog every day!"

"Why?" asked honest Molly.

"Because … never mind, just tell them."

And fortunately she did remember. The kennel staff were a little worried that Molly might not be able to manage such a young and potentially boisterous dog, but between us we convinced them otherwise, and five minutes later, papers and cheques signed, we were headed home, Tilly lying by my side on the back seat of the car as quiet as a mouse. What a lovely dog. And what a relief to have Mother be-dogged again; no more of the whingeing we had suffered during the past month. I was happier than I had been for weeks.

That evening I rang Sally to tell her the glad tidings, but she was out, so I left a message on her answer-phone; "Tilly Smith is in residence at Parc Bush." As soon as she got home, Sally rang Molly and said, "Can I speak to Tilly Smith please?"

In normal times Molly would have laughed and responded in kind, but now she just replied, "Who?" The memory was disappearing faster than we could keep up with.

The next day I called at Parc Bush, to find Molly out shopping and Tilly left all alone. The dog greeted me perfunctorily, then rushed out into the garden, sniffing as though on a trail, and looking hopefully at the gate.

"Ah, you want your new mum, don't you?" I said. How lucky we had been to find such a devoted dog.

And how wrong.

I waited for Molly to return from the shops and stood back to witness the effusive welcome from her new pooch. Tilly gave a slight wag and stood with a faraway expression in her eyes.

The next day she made her opinion of us perfectly plain. Molly, amazingly, set out to take her for a walk, but as soon as she was outside the gate, Tilly slipped her collar and set off up the road at a gallop, desperate to find the Lands End kennel maid whom she had imprinted as the alpha female. Molly set off in hot pursuit, accomplishing an incredible half mile before she managed to see someone coming the other way and gasp "Catch that dog!" which they did.

Was Tilly ever in disgrace! And did Sally and I ever hear about it! For the next three days, whenever we saw Molly she would complain that Tilly was the wrong dog for her. She was actually right, but after all our hard work getting a dog, and Molly's moans about not having one, this was not what we wanted to hear. Molly could still use the phone at this stage, and I was quite cross when I received an answer-phone message from her saying Tilly was "all over the place" and that she had not wanted a young dog. What did she want me to do about it? Send Tilly back to the dogs' home? I left yet another message on Sally's phone, this time threatening that I was going to commit matricide. I got one back from Sally, saying, "We'll keep the dog and stick *Mother* in a home!"

It was all very well laughing, but I was quite upset at the thought of Tilly not being the best dog for Molly, and although I kept burying the problem, it would keep disinterring itself. On Christmas Eve I was in tears.

I was not the only depressed one that season. Molly was supposed to come to us for Christmas lunch, but she phoned to cancel in the morning, saying she felt "yuck" and depressed. The weather was likewise. So John and I walked Tilly round the sheltered little valley of Poltesco in the rain and wind before coming back to Carmelin and dinner *à deux*.

On Boxing Day, Molly happily came to lunch with us and the Ellis family. Perhaps, I mused, it was only John and I who made her feel yuck and depressed! She stayed until 10 o' clock that evening, when Sally and Martin took her home. As belated Christmas Days go, it was a successful one.

Except that dear Tilly came too. She enjoyed herself on a long, wet walk with Sally's spaniel Clem, the pair of them returning soaked and muddy and being shut in the sherb to dry off, where they whined a dogs' chorus and scratched continuously at the door until we let them back in. Then they indulged in endless play-fighting which was noisier and more exhausting than any of us were used to since Wenna and Toana had grown up. Tilly homed in, like a food-seeking missile, on any plate left within striking distance and helped herself to mince pies, cake crumbs, marzipan, icing and whatever other yuletide offering she could find, including an exploratory lap at a glass of sherry. For her *pièce de résistance*, she piddled on the hall carpet. You might think of a Staffie as being a fairly small dog, but Tilly was a cross and the cross bit was, although officially whippet, more like lurcher. Big dog, big puddle. In the ensuing years the carpet has been shampooed at least five times, but, if you look carefully, the evidence of Tilly's first Christmas remains as a reminder and a lesson to us all. Listen to the CPN.

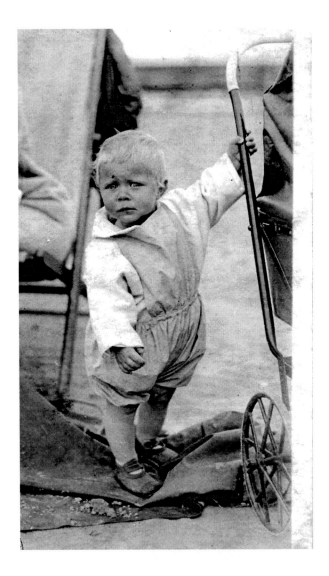

Molly aged 1

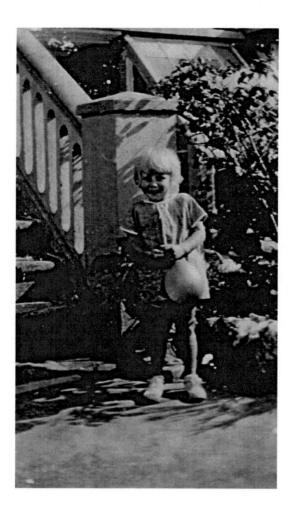

Did someone say Ice Cream?

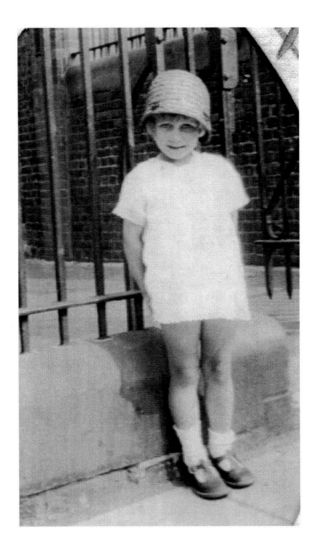

Outside Daddy's school

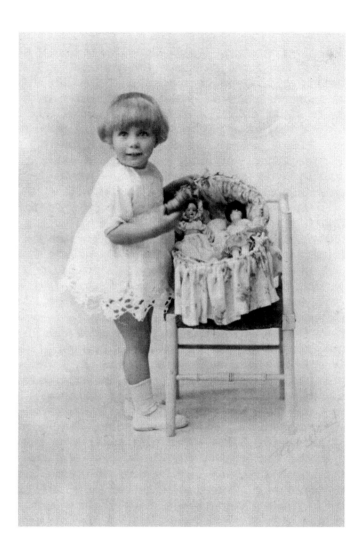

Molly and her dolly

CHAPTER 5

THE NEW MILLENNIUM

One of the strangest things about AD is how it takes one by surprise ("one" being the carer, as the sufferer for the most part cannot remember). There is, naturally, the steady and notorious decline in memory, but what is not so well known is that it affects other aspects of the sufferer's mental condition too, including mood and cognitive ability. You don't know what that last bit means? Nor did I, but it is a mixture of all the actual mental processes - awareness, perception, intuition, reasoning, to name a few; hence Molly's inability to do the crossword, the moments of depression, and the unreasonableness we encountered. However, at this stage we glossed over the latter and, like the world at large, worried just about Molly's forgetfulness.

2001 signalled the start of a new millennium (except for the mathematically challenged amongst the populace who thought that it had started on January 1st 2000) and a new era in the lives of Molly and her family. Since her illness had been diagnosed, we knew a little more of what to expect - emphasis on the word "little". The Redruth clinic staff were helpful and gave me a couple of printouts about AD generally - a Carer's Guide, The Seven Stages of Alzheimer's Disease (these days reduced to Four for reasons of economy), and Sundown Syndrome - all of which made pretty depressing reading - and any questions we asked were answered. But, as usual with any of the social services, resources were stretched and there was a limit to how much they could do. I also received a couple of free copies of the Saga magazine that year, so, aside from reading about Costa Fortune cruises, stair chairs, baths which you could step into wearing a swimsuit, chairs that project you out of your seat and across the room, plus some extremely dull regular columns, there was an excellent medical page. This would often include an AD related article, which was interesting even though many of the articles were about possible cures to take effect from 2020. I also discovered the AD website and various books on the subject. Thus began our education, and my AD antennae started to sprout.

It was amazing to read about the number of potential cures, palliatives and theories that were being discovered all the time. Dietary recommendations were endless; red foods (beetroots, tomatoes, water melons, berries - especially blueberries - peppers, red grapes, even red wine - yo!), green leafy veg, apples, sweet potatoes, beans, green beans, watercress, Brussels sprouts, carrots, pumpkin seeds, oats, wholemeal pasta and grains, "omega 3" rich eggs from chickens fed on flax seeds, oily fish - but be careful because so much fish is polluted, even if fresh from the sea - and dark chocolate (yo again!). Then there were the vitamins - E, C, B6, B12 and folic acid - and avoidance of chemicals, hydrogenated fats, fried foods, excess coffee and alcohol. The list continues to grow.

The food options sounded simple enough, and Sally and I put into effect what we could, but it was difficult when Molly was still doing her own shopping, consisting mainly of cake and the occasional sausage. She did buy apples but on their own these were pretty useless. I read about an Apples, Curry and Guinness cure which might be effective, but it was unclear whether one was supposed to take them separately or all at once, and the latter sounded more like a recipe for a DIY bubble bath.

More impressive sounding were the medical possibilities, from a simple daily aspirin, to a b-amyloid peptide vaccine; lithium (used as an antidepressant); neural precursors; the nerve growth factor (patient's skin cells injected into their brain), and even a drug used for Athlete's Foot. Tests are run continuously, and the laboratory mice are still working hard for us, so maybe the poor wee things will help scientists come up with a cure within the next few years.

In the meantime, our daily lives continued and we had to climb out of the gloom of a Cornish winter, accompanied this year by having to walk Tilly. Our chickens had come firmly home to roost, and the dog we had persuaded the kennels to let Molly adopt had to be exercised. After the December road-runner scare, Molly was not about to change the habit of a lifetime and take Tilly anywhere except the garden, so Sally and I took it in turns to take the dog for a proper walk, sometimes using the occasion to take Molly with us. This at least got Molly out of the house, exercised and engaged in some conversation and a change of scenery.

Tilly, however, was a nightmare. She had walked on the lead in such a ladylike fashion the day we adopted her that we thought she was fully trained. In reality she pulled like a steam engine and, if let off the lead, would rush off in several directions at once, causing Molly to go into a complete panic, and leaving Sally or me to perform concurrent duties of retrieving the dog and calming an agitated mother. In February, life became even more difficult when foot-and-mouth disease descended on the country. Fields were forbidden, and the wide open spaces of beaches were too risky with Tilly being so manic. So we had to walk her, on a lead, round the country lanes, picking up poop as we went. Lovely. We persevered, Sally bringing Clem and his mother, little old Beauty, and sometimes we could put Molly in charge of Beauty while we managed the younger dogs. But it wasn't much fun.

Then along came Hintza, the magnificent Ridgeback recently acquired by John's boys and their mum. Mum had suffered a knee injury and couldn't walk, so Hintza was given into Angus's and

Hamish's charge for a few weeks, and he came with them when they visited us. This lovable monster dog, weighing in at 7 stone, provided the first gleam of light in our sorry lives. He had to be walked, and there was no way he could remain attached to his lead unless the holders wished to be dragged across the countryside flat on their faces. So, as beaches were deemed foot-and-mouth free, we introduced Hintza and Tilly on Kennack Sands and, hearts firmly in mouths, let them both off the lead.

They went berserk. The pair of them rushed hither and yon and round in circles, across the beach, over the stream, into the woods, up and down hills, crashing through the undergrowth, chasing birds, rabbits and imaginary jungle beasts, barking and yapping themselves into complete hysterics. But, answering our prayers as well as our calls, Hintza came back when we yelled, and Tilly followed.

Needless to say, we had left Molly at home during this experiment, so when we put the exhausted, panting pooches into the car and delivered the girl back to her mum, we were able to report a successful venture.

"You didn't let her off the lead, did you?" enquired an anxious Molly.

"No way!" we assured her, crossing our fingers.

"That's all right then."

After that, John and I made it a regular task to collect Tilly from Molly and give her a good run. John, not really knowing how to handle the Molly situation, would wait patiently in the car, reading a book or listening to the radio while I was indoors doing whatever needed doing before bringing Tilly out. I sometimes felt guilty on his behalf, making him sit there, but I had to crush this feeling, as it vied with the guilt I felt at not giving Molly enough time. John didn't mind anyway; he preferred to relax with Radio-Something than to struggle making conversation with his mother in law. It had been bad enough when she was just reserved and shy; now that she was Alzheimic he didn't have a clue what to say. But he enjoyed the dog walking, and was very good with Tilly, teaching her to come when called, and instilling in her the difference between birds and cows, i.e., which of the two she was allowed to chase. She was a quick learner. She was also a lovable and loving dog and we both began to get very fond of her.

In spring of that year, we had good and bad news. The good was that Foot and Mouth was now under control and the public footpaths were open again. It was like being let out of prison. The bad news was that I sprained a ligament in my back very badly (yes, of course, digging in the garden. Is there a better way?) and was physically incapacitated to an extent I had never known.

Molly was a great help. I phoned to tell her my woeful tale, and she was most solicitous. Could she assist in any way?

"Well," I said, hesitantly, "I hardly like to ask, but I do have the garden to weed and the chalet to clean!"

This chalet is a little two-bedroom affair in our front garden that we let out on a long term basis, and the tenant had chosen this month, of all times, to move out. Not his fault, but there was a great deal of spring and post-tenant cleaning to be done, and I just couldn't cope.

"I'll come and lend a hand," said Molly as she so often did. She loved to be involved in family activities, even if it meant hard work, and she was a very efficient maid of all work.

"Will you really?" I asked. "That would be fantastic. I'll send John over to collect you."

Molly duly came and assisted. She was as willing as ever, and as long as I gave her a simple task, like mopping the floor, or wiping out cupboards, she could manage. I didn't let her work too long, but for nearly a week she and I laboured together just as we had in the old days, and we got the job done. Not only that, but she helped me in the garden too, weeding and potting-on plants, something that I could only do whilst lying flat on the grass on my tummy. This had occasioned many merry quips from anyone who spied me over the garden wall, mostly along the lines of what a nice relaxed way to do the gardening, but it most assuredly wasn't.

The doctor had told me that exercise would be good for me, particularly walking, and as soon as I was able to totter more than a few yards I used this excuse unashamedly. Molly was showing a gradual reluctance to partake of any physical exercise; we used to go swimming every week until the previous winter when she declared that she just "didn't feel right" in the water, and now she didn't want to come walking, saying that she was "Not very good at it any more." You would think, therefore, that she would be glad to have her dog taken for a run by someone else, but no, she did not like Tilly being absent for an hour. This was quite an obstacle to be overcome, for her maternal instincts on behalf of her dog were extremely strong, but, amazingly, I won by dint of appealing to her maternal instincts on behalf of me, which up until now had been the weaker. "Can I take Tilly for a walk? The doctor says it will be good for my back."

My wheedling won, and although Molly's memory was fairly rocky by this time, it seemed to sink in that I came along regularly and took Tilly out. I even ventured to reveal at last that I had let her off the lead. This was done in a very casual way, emphasising how good Tilly was, and that although she might walk ahead for a few yards, she would look back to check on me every few minutes. One day I even persuaded Molly to come with me.

"I don't know that I will be happy with her off the lead," she fretted.

"Oh, that's all right. Just pretend that she's *my* dog, not yours!" and Molly laughingly agreed. As we meandered slowly up the footpath from Poltesco, Til trotted off, and then looked back.

"Look!" I exclaimed. "See, she's making sure we're following her! Isn't she clever?" and with similar remarks made repeatedly throughout our walk, making sure it went into Molly's consciousness and stayed there, all was well.

At about this time, we were thrilled to welcome our Auntie Heather, Smithy's sister, from Canada for a fortnight's visit. She had last visited her sister-in-law two years before, and we warned her that Molly had changed quite a lot in that time. If she would rather stay with John and me, in our spare room, we would be quite happy to accommodate her. Heather was made of sterner stuff, though, and took up residence in Molly's spare room without a qualm.

Heather is a lovable nut case. Smithy always regarded her as his irritating little sister, and she tried his sibling patience to its limits. He would constantly be trying to calm her over-exuberant moods, prodding her with a finger, and with each prod saying, *"Don't - Get - Excited!"* and this became a family phrase which is in use to this day. Heather did have her merits though. When Smithy was in his teens and eager to impress the girls, he would coach his little sister in her role at the local swimming baths. Heather was instructed to go up behind any girl standing hesitating at the pool's edge and push her in, whereupon heroic Smithy would dive in and "rescue" the maiden. Whether kid sister was rewarded, or bribed, I don't know, but she probably enjoyed it anyway.

Heather and Molly enjoyed each other's company and always had done. The teenage Heather had been thrilled when her big soldier brother announced he had a steady girlfriend and when Heather badgered him to tell her about this new girl, Smithy replied, "When you meet her, you will realise that she is perfect." Heather was not disappointed, and she and the beautiful bride-to-be became instant friends. The friendship continued even when Heather and her husband emigrated to Canada, with letters flowing back and forth across the Atlantic for decades.

Letters, however, can never compete with human contact, so there was tremendous excitement when Heather announced her intention to visit us. To her credit, she coped perfectly with the new Molly, using just the right amount of chatter, laughter and patience, and seeming to have an innate understanding of the right thing to do. It was only when Sally and I got involved that we messed things up. We invited the ladies to a pub lunch and Heather agreed with alacrity.

"What about you, Molly?" I asked. "Would you like to come? You can bring Tilly - we're only going down to Cadgwith."

"No thanks," she replied. "And don't be too long, will you?"

"No, of course not," and off we dashed, complete with an eager

Tilly, diving into a wonderful hour of reminiscences, glasses of wine, and things with chips. Did I say hour? Well, maybe a little longer ... the landlord came across to us.

"Are you Molly's daughters?" he asked.

"Yes. How do you know that?"

"She's just rung. She wants her dog back."

We were amazed. Not that Molly wanted Tilly in preference to us, for that was typical, but we had not left her a phone number, and so she had had to trawl all through the Yellow Pages to find the Cadgwith pub. We walked back through the Cornish drizzle to Parc Bush, where Molly immediately took Tilly off to dry her, while Sally and I raided cupboard and fridge for coffee and cake. She and Heather and I carried on the party in the sherb, and it was a good half hour later when Heather remarked, "Where is Molly?"

We found her in the study, sitting on the floor, silently and moodily cuddling an extremely reluctant Tilly who could smell cake and wanted to join the party. We invited Molly to do the same but she frostily declined. She didn't say why, but the sad fact was obvious - she could no longer handle the excitement and bustle of a crowd of people having fun.

* * * * *

Molly was still keeping regular appointments with Dr B, taking the Mini Mental Test each time and coming through with colours, if not flying, at least attempting take-off. The Arricept seemed to be helping, steadying the decline in memory and keeping depression at bay for most of the time. However, there was bad news too.

"How long can we use this drug?" I asked.

"Oh, about twelve to eighteen months," replied Dr B. Molly had been taking it for six months already and my heart sank into my boots.

"And then what happens?"

"The disease takes it course."

Oh, great.

"So..." I hesitated, still in shock, and not knowing how to put this, "...how long ... have we got?"

"It's hard to say," said Dr B, "but on average five years until she won't be able to cope any longer."

All this was said in front of Molly, who said nothing and asked nothing. For all Dr B's consideration and cheerfulness, it did occur to me to wonder whether this "bedside manner" was quite kind to the client, and I might well have been as guilty as the doctor, but in reality I am pretty sure most of our conversation went over Molly's head.

Perhaps I should explain here our way of thinking in relation to how much we told Molly. Our policy was: As Little As Possible.

In this we were following our instincts. I might well be accused of being an ostrich, or turning another person into one, but I firmly believe that to inform a person how bad things are, when telling them can accomplish nothing, is immoral. When my father lay dying, and he asked Molly "Am I going to die?" she was incapable of saying anything other than the truth, but she watered it down as much as she could, answering, "It is possible, yes." When he asked the nurse the same question, the hard-hearted girl replied, "I am afraid so, Mr Smith, yes." Honesty - ten; bedside manner - nil. Had he asked me, I would have said, "Of course not! But it will be a long fight, and you have to be strong. Better rewrite your will, though, just in case!" This would have given him hope, would have added a touch of humour, and, when his body was finally in switch-off mode, he would have known nothing about it.

So, to tell my mother that she had an incurable and degenerative brain disease when she was intelligent enough to know what that meant, but not strong enough to cope with the inherent shock, grief, anger and bewilderment was, to me, unthinkable. Sally agreed. We took the Dulux approach and glossed over it big-time.

I have read other AD books on this issue, and opinions differ. Some say that, once the sufferer knows what she has to cope with, she can do so with forethought and understanding. Maybe so. But Molly, by the time her AD was diagnosed, even if she understood, was not in a state to remember it. Yes, she remembered that she was forgetful, but would she have remembered that she had AD? I doubt it. And, if she had, would she have felt better about the fate that awaited her? I doubt that even more. Far better to play the whole thing down, tell her that we were *all* getting absent minded, and deal with life as best we could. This is what we have always done, and I don't think we could have done it in any other way that would have kept Molly happier.

So, when Dr B and I discussed things in front of Molly, in a does-she-take-sugar mode, I don't think we were treating her like a second class citizen. Even if she had had any queries at the time, she would have forgotten the answers as soon as she walked out of the door.

There were other examples of her forgetfulness throughout this year. Dear old Beauty, Clem's mum, who had been on her last legs for months, took her final walk to the kennel in the sky that spring. Sally phoned to tell me the news, and said she had told Molly already. When I said to Molly two hours later, as we got home from shopping, "Isn't it sad about Beauty?" she had no idea what I was talking about. Neither could she recall having been shopping. When I asked if she had fed Tilly, she did not know. The brain cells were dying off faster than we could say goodbye and thank you.

John was at this time endeavouring to set up a new radio station for Cornwall, and was running a trial broadcast throughout a month of the summer. Because the station had to use a very low powered transmitter, any listener had to be halfway up the nearest hill in order to hear it. Our own house was too far down the valley, so I used to go and listen in Molly's dormer bedroom, one of the few places I could get reception, during the four weeks of the show. Molly forgot about the project every single time, and on each visit I had to explain why I was hanging myself and her radio out of the Velux window while I twiddled with the knobs on the set.

As evidenced by her daily jars, she forgot her blood pressure and Arricept pills three days running.

One morning she said she had forgotten to go shopping the day before, so I drove her down to Spar and helped her throw things in a basket. "I don't know why you're making me do this," she kept complaining, and I responded with suitably patronising noises, ignoring her protests because obviously she couldn't remember what she had just told me about forgetting to go shopping. When we got back to Parc Bush, I found a fridge and two cupboards full of her shopping from the day before. So she had actually forgotten that she *had* remembered to shop yesterday, and then remembered again when we were actually doing it. It didn't matter; at least she would have plenty to eat for the next day or two.

In spite of the constant additions to our list of surprises, we did manage to settle into some sort of pattern in dealing with Molly's life. Compared to what was to come, things were relatively simple at that time. Of course, even then, we were well aware that they could be worse, but what we didn't know was by how much, or when.

CHAPTER 6

THE CHRISTMAS LETTER

Christmas. Don't you just love it? Well, maybe the jury is still out on that. When we were children and all lived in London, Molly and Smithy did the whole number, inviting a perfect mix of family and friends, organising three sit-down meals and wall-to-wall entertainment. They would start planning in January, and, as I look back now, they could have done it for a living, so calm and professional were they. The party would spill over into Christmas Eve and Boxing Day, and the week afterwards would be spent accepting return invitations. The whole season was full of fun and jolliness. Then, when I was twenty, Molly and Smithy moved to Cornwall, the best thing that ever happened to our family in the long run, but our Christmas guests did not follow suit, and the parties got less and less exciting until they died out altogether. By 2001, it had become the tradition for Sally and Martin to spend Christmas day with Martin's parents, and although we all got together on Boxing Day, nothing could now match times past, and the season became largely a chore to be endured.

There were a few jobs I did still enjoy, however, and writing Christmas cards was one of them. For years, Molly had written a three page screed to add to her cards, only giving up a few years previously. But she and Sally and I still made a date each December to sit down together, writing our own cards and then sharing envelopes and postage where appropriate. It was a fun occasion with much chatter and laughter, cups of coffee and, of course, cake.

2001 was the last year that we did this. Sally and I had to talk Molly through the whole process, answering her confused questions for every single card. In former times, Molly had always written a little message, or at least put the name of the recipient, but we gave up on this. It was enough trouble for her to write three words.

"What do I write now?" she would ask.

"Just put *Love from Molly*", we would reply, and a few minutes' silence would reign while she laboriously wrote. Then ...

"What do I do now?" and we would hand her another card and repeat the instructions.

To the power of 100.

Sure, we all giggled our way through the process, but Sally and I looked at each other afterwards and shook our heads. Never again. We also made sure that Molly did not seal any of the envelopes, telling her that we wanted to put our own cards in later. It did not register with her that we had already done so, and that our true intent was to include a "Molly letter" of our own.

Writing my very first version of Molly's Christmas Letter was a long, and sometimes painful, process, but eventually I finished a two-pager. We imagined that many of her friends must have been wondering at her communications over the last few years, full of repetitions and oddities, jumping from one subject to another, much of it not the sort of thing you would tell anyone - for instance, the delivering and sorting of logs for the wood-burner; Molly went into screeds about this, unable to reason that it would have been of no interest to anyone, not even the log man. We also found out that she had come across several old letters that she had received - one going right back to 1984 - and had written and sent replies. So I stole her address book. Now my own letter explained what had been happening to Molly in the last few years, and one was tucked into each Christmas card envelope.

The following are just a couple of extracts:

It is a very strange business having Alzheimer's to deal with. Because it happens so gradually, you don't realise at first what is going on. Then, when the diagnosis comes, you think: OK, now what? The doctor and psychiatric nurses have been as supportive and helpful as their limited time allows. Even that seemed odd at first – my mother needing psychiatric help? But indeed she does. The strangest thing is that she seems perfectly normal for so much of the time. And she can manage most of her day-to-day life with our help. This has gone on for so long, and may continue to do so, that we are lulled into complacency. Then occasionally we are jolted out of this; for instance, the other day Molly was in the garden and said to Sally that she didn't know whose garden it was. So we know this sort of thing will continue to happen and there won't be a happy ending, but we muddle along as best we can. As for what the ending will be, I only hope it won't be Molly living in an old folks' home not knowing her knitting from her knickers, but we shall just have to see.

I am telling you all this, not to paint a thoroughly black picture, but to prepare you in case you get in touch with Molly, and I hope you will. She is not "loony" as she puts it, just forgetful. She is the same old Molly, with a sharp wit, observation and sense of fun, and indeed it has seemed to us at times that these senses have actually been increased, the brain making up in these areas for what it has lost in others. One common symptom in AD patients is a heightened sense of colour and shape, and Molly definitely demonstrates this. Her kitchen is a veritable florist's shop of flower arrangements, even at this time of year, in all sorts of vases and containers, and she is constantly pointing out shapes and shades she has noticed. Not only that, but funnies in writing too – misprints and peculiar expressions on packets, jars and bottles for instance, such as "Best consumed before end", which had her in stitches. So there is still a helluva lot up above!

By the way, if you do get in touch with Molly, please do not use the term "Alzheimer's", and do treat the subject lightly. If she says she is forgetful, just say, "Yes, me too," and tell her a story of how you walked into a … what was it? Oh yes, a room, and looked for … um … you know the sort of thing.

Within days I was overwhelmed with phone calls and letters. People had indeed been wondering about Molly, and were so very pleased that Sally and I were taking care of her. Although I had intended the letter to be merely factual, writing it had brought a lump to my throat, and the responses did likewise. How good to know that friends and distant relations cared about her so much. And a bonus for me was getting in touch with people who had been grown-ups when I was a child, whom I had never got to know very well. Now I chatted to them as equals, and learned such a lot about them. The only danger I had to avoid was promising to keep in touch as Molly had done. She was such a good correspondent that she would sit down at her tripewriter, as she called it, and bash out a response to any letter she received almost on the day she received it. Now my replies would be once a year.

Cards, letters and phone calls also came directly to Molly. The phone calls were a little awkward, as she could not retain a subject long enough to have a conversation, but as long as the caller was happy to do most of the talking, Molly could certainly appreciate and enjoy the call.

The responses calmed down after a month or two, then, out of the blue, came a ghost from our past. While sorting through a pile of papers at Molly's, Sally found a letter going back years, from a friend of Molly and Smithy's in the local sub-aqua club. They had both been enthusiastic skin divers for some years in the 1960's, and had made very many good friends, but there was a special core including a young guy called Adrian Davies. The only things I remember about him at the time were that he had a shock of ginger hair and didn't seem to like kids much. This did not deter my ten year old brother Royce, who plagued him constantly, but Adrian and I had nothing at all in common and I rarely even spoke with him. A couple of years later he introduced his girlfriend, Laurel, to us all, and she became part of our lives. She remains so to this day, even though she and Adrian broke up decades ago. He later went to America where he met and married Jill, and they have been a devoted couple all these years since.

Although his details did not appear in Molly's address book, nor on her Christmas card list, Adrian's letter carried his address, and

Sally and I wondered if we should now send him a Christmas letter too. We eventually decided - why not? and sent off the letter, with a covering one to remind Adrian who we were.

He had not forgotten. The phone rang at Carmelin one evening and it was Adrian, calling from America. He remembered us all, and, although sad to learn about Molly, had been very happy to hear from us. Strangest of all was the fact that he had a similar problem in his family, Jill's mother, who also suffered from AD. So we compared notes, had a bit of a chat about old times, and prepared to say goodbye. Then I said, as an afterthought, "If you want to write to Molly, send me an e-mail and I will pass it on to her."

Within days I received an e-mail from him, starting with a polite

> *Thanks for putting me/us on the newsletter list, and of course, news of Molly, however sad, is welcome.*

But lapsing very soon into what I was to learn was typical Adrian style...

> *If there is any good at all in this, it is that she herself is not going to know what is going on. Hard for me to imagine, anyway; my most vivid memory of Molly is of her in a bikini on a Cornish beach!*

Adrian was right; Molly remained in blissful ignorance of her plight for the most part - as, no doubt, she would have been of Adrian drooling over her in her swimwear. He and I have now been in touch for over six years, and more e-mails have flowed back and forth between me and this guy (and *sometimes* Jill, his wife) than almost anyone I know. In the struggle of looking after an AD patient, it is good to have support, and we seem to have provided that for each other and our respective families. Indeed, we have become an extension of each other's family. In different circumstances, the elderly ladies might well have met and become friends, but at the very least, their offspring have now done so.

So, Jill's mum. Does she have a name? I imagine so, but I can't remember Adrian ever using it. His first e-mail, sent in February 2002, ended with the following words:

> *Gotta go, because I am supposed to be cooking supper, while Jill is down the road with her mum, the Pob [Poor Old Bugger], and I am getting a bit short of time.....*

Using this affectionate shorthand, we have referred to her as Pob ever since.

CHAPTER 7

AN E-MAIL FROM AMERICA

Sally and I, mutually supportive, seemed to be managing. But Jill, although she had Adrian's 100% support, would find a harder road ahead of her. For the first few years of our correspondence, it was always Adrian who wrote and sent the emails, apart from a short one from Jill at the beginning, along the lines of "Hi! I'm Jill, and I have no problem with you writing to my husband! I'll send something myself as soon as I get the time." Well, Jill had a full time job as a tax advisor, which took her out of the house all day, whereas Adrian worked from home and could at least bash out a few lines on the computer in a spare moment. Much later, Jill wrote me a long, long letter, of which the section below gives some of the background to Pob's dementia:

> I believe it would be impossible for anyone who has never met us to appreciate the depth of my feelings. Mum was a really fun lady, with tremendous inner strength. After my father passed away, 33 years ago, she was a young 58 year old widow. She relocated to be near myself and Adrian. She always considered him to be her second son, and they got along well. We found a house just two blocks from ours, where she has lived for over twenty years. We included her in our social life and vacations. She never interfered, was unselfish, loving, supportive and funny. Her presence enhanced our lives. Three days after her 85th birthday, she led us in a climb to the top of Diamond Head in Hawaii!
> During the week of our arrival back home, she fell in her bathroom and hit her head. She seemed OK, but a couple of evenings later said she had been sleeping a lot during the day, so we took her along to the hospital, and the doctor verified that she had concussion. We were given the name of a neurologist, and told to make an appointment if she did not recover. She did recover, as far as we could tell. And since she had been having periods of forgetfulness for some time, we were not too concerned. However, about a year later, we finally made the appointment with the Neurologist. The neurologist confirmed that she had Alzheimer's. So then, finally, it dawned on me that I was losing my mum.

It was sad to read a story so similar to Molly's - Pob's knock on the head having, apparently, the same effect as Molly's blackouts. But it had not occurred to me, or to Sally, to feel that we were *losing* our mother, and I wondered why we were not equally devastated by Molly's problem. Perhaps she was not so far along Dementia Drive as was Pob, but was *our* approach too light-hearted? I did not wonder for long. The answer was an emphatic No. We were doing what seemed natural to us, being sympathetic but realistic, smoothing her path through life whilst continuing on our own, avoiding confrontation but sometimes gently teasing, and at every available opportunity seeing the funny side.

If Sally and I do sometimes feel guilty at how much we laugh, I can blame this on my mother too. She, and indeed her own mother, our Nan, found the funny side in nearly everything. I remember my father remarking on this a few weeks before he died, saying to Molly, "You laugh at everything, don't you?" and he meant this as a compliment. As I see it, anything that gets us through this ghastly situation is OK, and, if we can get Molly to join in, which so often we do, that is a bonus. So, to quote from one of Molly's favourite operas, *Ridi, Pagliacco* - the smiling clowns in this case being Sally and I - and, most important, don't feel any guilt at your laughter. Does it harm the patient? No. Does it help the carers? Yes. Well, then. *Vesti la giubba.* (Go look it up; it will help to exercise your brain cells.)

Adrian's approach to Pob's difficulties (poblems?) was as light-hearted as ours to Molly's, but again this did not mean he did not care, for he did, desperately. For his ma in law of whom he was so fond, and for his wife, whose suffering he had to witness. Sales of bourbon, he said, had reached an all time high at his local liquor store. Still, he was encouraged by some of my more wry emails to send funny stories of his own. He sent a photo of his mother in law, with the following ...

> Since you asked about Pob, here she is. We also have another name for her, "the old bat". She still has her personality, and we find ourselves wondering when exactly this dementia started. She has always made the most dippy statements, as far back as I can remember, and even now anyone who talks to her probably will not notice anything wrong if the conversation is short. But one has only to ask what year it is ("1928") or what town we live in ("Dartford, Kent"), or hear her use anachronisms from her early days in the UK, like "quid" and "bob" instead of cents and dollars, and it becomes painfully obvious. She has always been such a funny old girl. So, although all the doctors and psychologists might know a helluva lot, none of them have ever met an old bat before.

I wasn't too sure of that! But the next paragraph demonstrated Pob's unique personality to perfection.

One of her WW2 accomplishments was to date Ian Smith, later prime minister of Rhodesia, (now Zimbabe, not spelt right, but who cares?) who flew a Hurricane. One day, some years ago, I was up on the roof, fixing something, and she called out to me, "Be careful!" This was so obvious and unnecessary, that it annoyed me, so when I climbed back down I told her not to talk such nonsense. "What about all those airmen you dated in the war?" I asked. "They were flying fighter planes and bombers and doing parachute landings. Did you tell them to Be Careful?" She looked me straight in the eye and replied, "Only when they were in my bed!"

The really rotten thing about all this is that she has been such a loveable old stick, and on top of it all, she is Jill's mum, and Jill is the one going through the real hell. There is a lot to be said for a damned good heart attack. However, this is getting a bit philosophical, so I am going to sign off, and pour another whiskey.

Some time in the next couple of years, we are going to come and visit you, and the four of us can head off to Royce's pub and get pissed.

And indeed they did, but that is another story.

CHAPTER 8

THE DAY JAR VIEW

The New Year of 2002 started like most in Cornwall; theoretically mild, but with wet-and-wind chill factors making it thoroughly unpleasant to be anywhere but indoors, preferably under a duvet. But nothing deterred Sally or me from our daily walks with Tilly, and, if the weather was not too wild, Molly would come with me. I learned to avoid any steep climbs or cliff path walks, because, although she was quite fit, she was very unsure of herself in such places. This vertiginous aspect perhaps explained her "not good any more" protestations, so I directed our walks to safer places, an amble through the softly green and beautiful Poltesco Valley, sheltered from the winds, or across a sandy beach. One day I took her to the wide expanse of Kennack Sands, where she had not been for probably thirteen years, and we headed up the woodland trail behind the beach, scene of Tilly and Hintza's first encounter but a completely new walk for her.

"Oh, I've been here before, haven't I?" she remarked brightly.

"Yes, we came to the beach for a swim one summer evening years ago," I replied.

"No, I mean in the woods."

"Oh, the woods. Oh yes, we've been here lots of times." Funny how easy it was becoming to lie through my teeth, but better that than upsetting her and robbing her of any confidence she still had.

Soon after that, we were in a newly opened Mullion café, and she "recognised" it as soon as we walked in. In February we made a visit to her dentist, and were sitting in the waiting room, catching up on the last century's National Geographics, when Molly nudged me, pointing to a picture of an old railway station and poking her finger at it enthusiastically. "I've been there!" she exclaimed.

"Oh? Where is it?" I asked.

"In Wales, it says."

Wales? This was so unexpected that my normal porky mode temporarily crashed, and I could only reply truthfully that she probably hadn't actually been there, but that it was maybe similar to one she had visited.

Half a minute later, the same magazine, and a picture of a crowd of men.

"I've met those men!" she stated.

I continued in the same vein. "Mother, they're in Wales too, so I don't think you did!" and we chuckled together. She could always cope with being potty, as she called it, if we made light of it.

The dentist visit had been instigated because Molly had lost her plate containing one lonely little plastic canine peg, but the good news was that I had forewarned Molly of the appointment, and she had remembered. So, when the dental nurse phoned her to ask if we could make it to an earlier appointment, Molly immediately rang me to convey the message. This was six years ago, as I write, but it seems inconceivable now that she could once have managed to do something even that simple. She could also, at that time, talk about dentures, although she could not find the right word. Thus she explained,

"It'll be much better when I have ... those things you put in your mouth and take out again."

I considered this, then asked, "Do you mean bananas?"

We were still giggling when we were called into the surgery.

I had slipped a letter to the receptionist earlier explaining Molly's condition, so by the time I accompanied my mother into the surgery (what a role reversal *that* was!) the pleasant lady dentist was well aware of the situation. Saying that the less trauma Molly experienced the better (with which Molly and I fervently agreed), she just replaced a front crown and advised leaving the plate out completely. This left a gap in Molly's smile, but was better than the alternative, since she was constantly forgetting to take the plate out to clean it, and this was creating mild gingivitis. She soon lost it anyway, and I found it some months later, grinning at me from a drawer in her bedroom. I left it there for several months until it disappeared completely to who knows where.

Leaving the dental surgery, we did a little shopping, Molly gleefully immersing herself in the delights of the Mullion schlock shop, where she bought a pretty little glass ship complete with delicate filigree rigging. Then it was coffee and cake at the café, plus a few goodies to take home, before setting off back to Parc Bush. Unloading all the bags onto the worktop, I bent down to make a fuss of Tilly who was dancing a fandango on the kitchen floor, trying to grab my attention and my wrist. Molly turned to the cake.

"Ooh yum!" she grinned, helping herself to a large bite of treacle flapjack and picking up one of the other packages. "Whose is this?"

I looked up. It was the little box containing the ship, which she had bought not an hour before. Trying to keep the amazement out of my voice, I answered, "That's what you bought at the gift shop. It's yours."

"Is it? I don't remember."

Molly proceeded to unwrap it. "Oh yes," she said, "I remember that!" as it all came flooding back. Nowadays it wouldn't.

It is strange, but when I think back a few years to the late 90's when she coped so well with everything on her own, I can scarcely believe it, so quickly have we become used to the present circumstances. It is her previous state of capability that now seems odd. We have done our best to adapt to this situation as quickly as possible, and also to glean from it whatever positive things we can, and it is remarkable that there are any positives at all, but there are. And the fact that nothing can be changed means that there is no point in getting frustrated about it. So we have always tried to be sensible and kind, and, as I have stressed elsewhere, to appreciate the humorous aspect. Just occasionally, this was difficult.

One afternoon, when I had had two horrendous days at my school secretarial post, and faced yet more before the end of the week, I rushed over to Molly's, in between two loads of washing, to do Tills and pills duty. The first would be easy, and Tilly greeted me with her usual enthusiasm. Molly was less keen.

"Here we are," I said, trying to inject a note of gaiety into my tired voice. "A treat for you! It's pill time."

"I've already had them," she said, wandering off to poke at a drooping flower arrangement.

"No, you haven't," I argued stupidly. "Look, they're still in the Wednesday pot."

"Well, I can't help that. Someone must have changed the label."

Grinding my teeth, I dropped the subject, and went out to put Tilly in the car. I came back in and started afresh.

"Oh, look! You haven't had your pills. Shall we do it now and get it over with?"

"No, I *have* had them. I don't want any more."

Forgetting all my resolutions, I just got cross.

"Honestly, Mother, we are just trying to help you, but you make it so difficult for us!"

"No, I don't."

"Yes, you do!"

"No, I ..."

But I was not listening. "I'm going to walk the dog. See you later!" and I left her to the flower arrangements and stomped off before the conversation degenerated further. It was poor Tilly who had to bear the slammed car door and beating of fists on steering wheel. So don't feel bad if this happens to you (just don't do it in the Alzheimic presence). We are not saints, but sometimes we expect ourselves to act as though we were.

On the other side of the Atlantic, other saints were at work, and I received the following e mail from Adrian.

> *Jill took her mum to the neurologist this morning, hoping to get a change of medication because the drug Pob has been taking (Exelon) has been having no apparent effect. I have always thought that Alzheimer's was a slow decline, but the old*

girl's deterioration has galloped in the past few months. It looks as though there is nothing that can be done but for us to look after the old girl, and try to make her life as comfortable as possible for as long as she lasts. Jill and I have always made a pretty good team, so I am sure we will handle it. We are both agreed that we will do anything we can to keep her out of a nursing home. American nursing homes are little more than carcass warehouses. Like most other people, I fear death, but there are things that I fear a helluva lot more.

On a lighter note, his next e mail mused...

Pob has always said and done the flakiest things imaginable, so I suppose that is what deceived us and we didn't see what should have been obvious. Several years ago, she wanted an electric lawn mower, so we got her one. But she never used it, because she couldn't fathom out how to plug it in. The first time, she was trying to plug it into the garden hose, and in all those years never did learn how to operate it.

It was years since Molly had used a lawn mower. She had several but, with typical dementia-type unreasonableness, she preferred to cut the large lawn bit by bit with the garden shears. On the one occasion I did organise the local gardening chap to take his mower to Parc Bush and do the job, Molly showed him no gratitude at all and in fact was so rude to him that he finished the job in double quick time, left and never returned. However, Molly was still interested in flowers and plants, so on a sunny June day I took her on a visit to a garden at a gorgeous old rectory at The Lizard. I had never visited this garden, and I knew Molly had not so much as set foot in it, but she "recognised" it all.

I don't often listen to the radio, but fate switched it and me on concurrently soon after the above visit and I caught a programme about people with brain damage. In particular they were discussing *déjà vu* symptoms, the very thing that Molly seemed to have been experiencing. One man was so bad that he was "remembering" things every few minutes. The phenomenon was partly explained by the fact that a different part of the brain takes over, registering the present as though it were the past. I mentioned this to Amie, our new and rather lovely CPN, and she was interested but, as with most AD symptoms, could shed no light on it. Sally and I quickly got used to Molly's "memories", and simply humoured her. Maybe, if you are losing your real memory, a false one is the next best thing.

This false friend was a convincing one, to Molly anyway. She and I were putting away some linen in her spare bedroom one day, and she pointed out the bedside chest with its missing drawer handle.

"Look at that!" she said crossly. "That woman who stayed here took it off! Wasn't that nasty?"

Today's answer would be, "Oh dear! The things some people will do! I wonder what she did with it?" but at that time I answered matter-of-factly that only our Auntie Heather had stayed in this room.

"It wasn't Heather; I know Heather," she said - and this in itself was heartening. "It was an old woman with white hair."

"Well, it was probably you looking in the mirror!" And, ruefully, she concurred. I had no clue what this was about, but then I had just as little clue how AD could affect the brain of someone who still seemed, quite often, quite reasonable.

* * * * *

Appearances could also deceive doctors. Because of her recent fall, Pob was due for a medical check-up.

> We took her to see the neurologist last Friday, and, because of her fall a while back, he gave her a lecture on the importance of using a walking stick - which she has always refused to do. Jill and I stood and watched him doing this, both simultaneously thinking "You ******g idiot, don't you, of all people, realise that one minute from now she will have forgotten everything you are saying, and we will not even have left this building before she has forgotten that she has even been to a doctor?"
>
> Anyway, once again "the luck of the devil" was as strong as ever and she seems to be relatively undamaged. If you or I were to fall, we would try to save ourselves somehow but Pob freezes up and topples over just like a falling tree. Looking after her is a bit like driving in very heavy traffic; everything ticks along ok but it takes only a second's inattention for something serious to happen.

I could only be glad that things were nowhere near that bad with our Molly.

CHAPTER 9

HUSBANDS

One day, Sally, Molly and I were all having a cup of coffee in Parc Bush kitchen, whilst Molly rummaged through a box of old cards she had recently found. One of them was an anniversary greeting from Smithy. There had been a time in our parents' lives, about twenty years before, when they had temporarily split up. A combination of menopausal moodiness, stress induced by trouble at t'mill, and general lack of understanding resulted in their treating each other rather badly, and Smithy left the Cornish valleys to reside once more in London. He eventually realised the error of his ways and returned to Molly, and she welcomed him back with open arms, but had apparently never entirely forgiven him, or forgotten this period of her life. His departure from the marital rails was what had lodged in her remaining memory.

She looked at the card for a moment with its customary *"All my love, Darling, from Smithy"* and thrust it back in its box.

"Huh!" she grunted. "I don't know what happened to *him*, and I don't care."

Sally and I exchanged glances, and Sally took it upon herself to explain, "Mother, he died."

"Did he?" responded Molly. "Oh, that's all right then."

Sally and I couldn't help it; we shrieked with laughter; and Molly joined in. We knew that Smithy would also have found it amusing, and could imagine his wry smile up in his Heaven, but Sally and I reflected later how distressing this sort of thing could be if it happened too often. There was little danger of that, however. Within a few months, Molly did not even recognise pictures of her late husband, and that was even worse.

As for me, I was about to have a new husband. July was upon us and, with it, the wedding of the year. After nearly four years of living together, John and I had finally got around to tying the nuptial knot. It was to be a small affair, but even so there was much preparation in the months beforehand. On the actual day, therefore, I felt justified in excusing myself from all dog and Mother duties, and Sally amiably agreed to do whatever was necessary. At this period Molly's fashion sense was well on the decline, and she could seldom see any good reason for putting on her glad rags if she didn't feel like it. In case she didn't on The Day, we had a dress rehearsal the week before, while she was in a good mood, seeing what clothes in the wardrobe still fitted both herself and the occasion. We chose a very pretty blue and pink two-piece, and I lent her back the white woollen jacket she had given me ten years before. We are not fashion icons down here in the country, but we think we have exceedingly good taste so it doesn't matter.

Being busy and preoccupied on the wedding day (funny, that ...) I had no chance to ask Sally if all had gone well chez Ellis/Smith, but later learned from daughters Wenna and Toana that they were really cross with their mum for refusing to let them do her hair in a special way. But poor Sally, after walking Tilly, which was the easiest job of the day, had had to spend forever getting Molly dressed and ready, and she had no time to do anything for her own ensemble but grab her dress (freshly ironed by a guest!), throw it on, run a comb through her hair, apply her lippy, and get to the register office on time.

In the middle of all that, my brother Royce, having left his wife Patti in charge of the inn, arrived at Sally's on his motorbike, dressed in his leathers, and needing somewhere to change into more gentlemanly attire, and thus added to the chaos. All was eventually accomplished, however, and the cavalcade set off for town. Molly behaved impeccably, sitting quietly during the ceremony taking it all in, as far as we could tell, and later on chatted with my friend Shirley at the lunchtime garden party. Both the ladies were fussy about their food, and would not dream of trying any of the savoury delicacies and exotic salads, so I raided the fridge for bread and Quorn, and stood at the kitchen worktop in my finery making sandwiches for them. They happily ambled off up the garden, balancing plates and glasses of OJ (teetotallers as well as fuss-arses), and were seen sitting on the patio happily chatting away while they munched. One would hardly have known there was anything wrong with Molly.

Her moment of glory came when we cut the cake. Not only could she indulge her staple diet, but she made herself really useful, handing it round to all and sundry, and although she didn't remember any names, and possibly no faces either, it didn't really matter. She got smiles and thank-you's galore, the atmosphere was jolly, and she enjoyed her afternoon. She was taken home later to spend the rest of the day quietly with Tilly, having declined the invitation to the evening party. She made her dog the excuse, and a few years later we found the draft of a letter she had written for her formal reply. She was always very proper.

Dear Jane
Thank you for your information. I have decided that I cannot be with you on the great day. I wood *would!!! have to be away from the dog for a long time so I would have to leave her alone or put her in the Kennels. I would not like leaving her. In fact I do not have many (or any - mostly!) visitors - so dog is the one I talk to mostly. Yes, I know I'm batty!*
I hope that you have a very happy day and that the sun shines.
Happy days, Love from Molly.

It appeared that Molly had intended to refuse even the daytime invitation, but happily had been persuaded otherwise. She seemed, on the surface, so well able to cope in a social situation that, apart from a very few people, mostly family, none of our wedding guests had any idea that she was suffering from AD. We did not deliberately hide the fact, and in fact assumed that people absorbed the information gradually, but it was apparently a shock to some. One day John got a phone call from Tess and John, long standing friends of John's and mine, and Tess asked him if we were doing anything that evening.

"I don't think so," replied John. "Why do you ask?"

"Well, John and I are going to the pictures in Helston and wondered if you and Jane would like to come too."

"That sounds great! I'll just check with Jane, and get back to you. By the way, what's the film?"

"It's 'Iris'."

"Oh!" said John and was quiet for a moment. "That's the one about Iris Murdoch, isn't it?"

"Yes, that's right," said Tess. "It's supposed to be very good."

"Yes, I'm sure it is, but, if you don't mind, Tess, I think we'll pass on that one. It's a bit too close to home."

"What do you mean?"

"Well, because of Jane's mum."

"What about her?"

"She has Alzheimer's. Didn't you know?"

"I had no idea!" said Tess. "Oh dear, you must think me so insensitive!"

Of course, we thought no such thing, and in fact I would not have minded seeing the film. John, in protective mode, had not even mentioned Tess's call to me, and I didn't find out until years later.

A month or two after our wedding, there was a shock in store for another friend, Olive, who came over from Australia to visit. She was actually my paternal grandfather's second wife, and when grandfather died, she had emigrated to Australia, starting a new life for herself. But she kept in close touch with us, and visited every so often. We had kept her up to date with Molly's illness, but, encouraged by Heather's visit two years before, reckoned that Molly was not so bad that she couldn't cope with Olive staying there for a few days. Knowing that Molly might need reminding who Olive was, I arranged to be at Parc Bush when Olive arrived, so that I could effect re-introductions. Something delayed me, however, and I drove up to the gates just in time to see Olive rummaging in her car boot with a worried frown.

"Oh!" she said, looking up and seeing me. "Thank goodness you've come! I don't know what to say to Molly! She's sitting there not saying a word, and I've completely run out of conversation. I was just looking for some photos to show her instead."

We went back indoors together, and the photos were duly produced for Molly, who really enjoyed them. This occasion was another wake-up call for me; just because I still found it easy to chatter with Molly, I should not have assumed it would be the same for someone who had not seen her for such a long time. Once she had got over the initial shock, Olive actually coped very well, and she was able to take Molly out and about with her, although preferably with either Sally or myself too!

As well as her tendency to flower-arrange anything in sight, another of Molly's new hobbies was hoarding things. She had always been a squirrel in that regard, but now she collected all sorts of packaging, including foodstuff wrappings which would be carefully washed, dried, and put back in the fridge. I had noticed the state of her fridge some weeks earlier, and at every opportunity I would remove the odd wrapper, stuffing it in my pocket when Molly was not watching, but it was difficult to do much as she always seemed to be hovering. If I so much as suggested throwing out a piece of paper, never mind removing a moribund bunch of flowers, she would protest vehemently. Now, however, was my big chance. One day when Olive and Sally had taken Molly out to tea, I moved in with the black plastic sacks. First I emptied the fridge and put all its contents on the floor so that I could take a photo, since no-one would believe it, including myself in a few years' time. I then stuffed the rubbish into two sacks, hustled them out to the car and crammed them into the boot before Molly made a reappearance.

This was the beginning of the Big Clean Up, and whenever Sally or I had the chance - perhaps when Molly had headed for the shops - we would home in on the fridge and kitchen cupboards, to empty them of their magpie-esque collections, dashing outside every so often to look down the road and make sure Molly and her trolley were not heading home - she walked at a rate of knots and could be back at Parc Bush before we knew it. This clearing out was in addition to checking the flower arrangements and disposing of the dead ones and dirty water, as we had been doing for ages when her back was turned, and gradually things began to look tidier.

Until autumn. Just outside the kitchen door was a beautiful eucalyptus tree, which Molly had grown from seed and nurtured lovingly for years. Its greeny-purple leaves would flutter down any time from October onwards, sprinkling the ground with perfectly formed oval shapes which were quite irresistible to Molly. She would collect every single one, bring it indoors and arrange it, along with the flowers, bread and butter, banana slices, toffee papers and pieces of cheese. These arrangements would go the way of the rest of the rubbish, but as soon as I threw out one hundred eucalyptus leaves, another thousand would follow. This went on for years, every autumn, but during the last year, Sally took to throwing them not into the rubbish, but back onto the lawn, reasoning that picking them up again would give Molly something to do, and keep her from meddling in more important things. This worked like a charm for a time, but these days she just looks at the leaves on the ground and tuts at the mess.

Molly was always happy when fiddling around with things, and needed no better entertainment than pottering around her home and garden, with just the occasional treat of a trip somewhere with Sally or myself. Across the Atlantic, however, Pob was a much more seasoned traveller, and another story beamed its way to my computer screen.

Another real problem for Pob is her vertigo. Plane travel is out of the question, so for our holidays we drove to Florida, and spent a couple of superb weeks in a condo. Pob enjoyed it enormously; memory loss or not, she is still talking about it, and asking when are we going back there! While we were away, we noticed that she always ate a good breakfast, although at home she never bothered. Don't know if it is our imagination, but we got the impression that she improved. There is no doubt that she remembers damned nearly everything about Florida. It could have been the stimulation of doing something different, but Jill and I have now adopted the habit of cooking breakfast for her. As she lives just down the road from us, Jill drops it in on her way to work.

This was happy news, and I was amazed that Pob could actually remember anything about the trip. Molly sure as heck would not have been able to do so. But sadder news followed, and a second "trip" was not so fortuitous.

Pob fell in her kitchen, and this time her usual luck was not with her; she broke her femur. We got her to hospital and she was operated on the next day. She then spent three weeks in a re-hab facility. A broken leg usually means curtains for oldies here, same as UK. But our Pob is in very good physical condition. The surgeon said that he had seen patients in their forties with worse bone density and muscle tone than she had. Too bad her brain is not in the same league.

However, you know this saying "The operation was a success, but the patient died"? Well, an American operating theatre is probably the best place to have an operation. But the after care is shit. Poor communication, too few nursing staff - badly trained and over-worked - can result in drugs being given too early, too late, not at all, or the wrong dosage.

This sounded, sadly, an all too familiar story, echoing what happens too often in the UK. But the effect on Pob was sadder still.

The surgeon who fixed Pob's leg refused to use a general anaesthetic, and avoided certain pain-killers because they would accelerate the AD deterioration. However, after an operation the surgeon goes out of the picture and the recovery is handled by whoever is on duty. Well, the doctor attending Pob had not thoroughly read her file and he prescribed one of the very pain-killers that the surgeon had avoided. One cannot really blame the doctor, since he had to see as many patients as possible, each one meaning a fee of a couple of hundred bucks for little more than saying Good Morning, and you can't hang around too long at that kind of cash can you? But the drugs worsened her condition immediately. She was on another planet, hallucinating like hell, and we had to take it in turns to stay at the hospital because we were the only two people she would co-operate with. However, although Jill and I didn't feel too kindly towards this gentleman, the brutal truth is that his incompetence actually did us a favour because Pob is now a lot closer to letting us off the hook than she would have been if this mistake had not been made.

Adrian was indeed being brutal in his honesty, but one sometimes has to face facts in this battle, to know when one is winning and when losing, and whether lost ground can be recovered, or if a new path has to be sought in caring for one's loved one. The new path for Adrian and Jill was a house move.

Now that Pob is home again, we have moved in with her to get her over the worst of it, but she seemed to get even more confused for a while, not even knowing who we were - for a while she thought I was her husband. A bit un-nerving that was! ("I'll take death, M'lud"). I can think of a couple of women whom I would really love to suffer from that delusion, but Pob ain't one of them.

Several decades previously, of course, Molly certainly would have been!

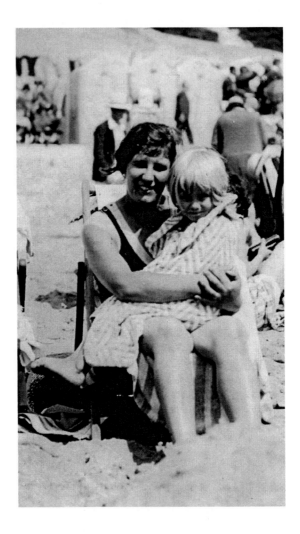

Cuddles with Mum on
Bournemouth Beach

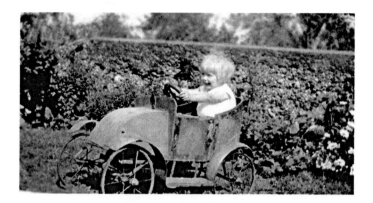

First driving lesson

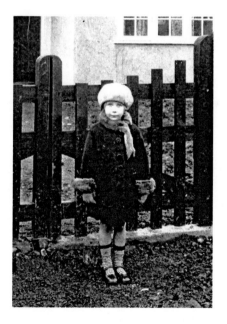

First day at school

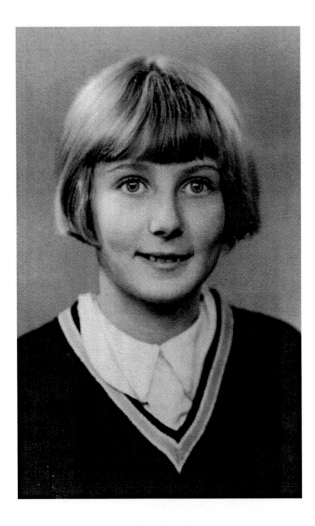

Eltham High School pupil
c1937

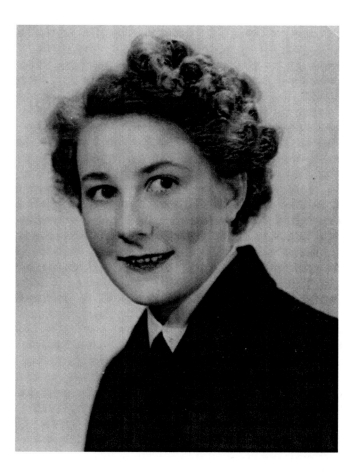

WREN
Molly Pembroke
1944

CHAPTER 10

THE PLOT THICKENS

It was now well over six years since my "Oh, Christ" moment in Molly's sherb, and, all things considered, we were doing pretty well. Molly was still living alone, doing her own washing, shopping and feeding. I won't say cooking, because by now she had forgotten that the cooker was for anything other than storing kitchen utensils (inside) or arranging flowers (on top). In former years she had fried sausages and chips every single night; not very nutritious, but she had made up for it at lunchtime with the few fruits and salad items that she could stomach ... celery, tomato, apple ... chocolate. Now she, and dear Tilly, survived mostly on a diet of bread and cake. In spite of this, Molly remained as slim as ever, but we were concerned about Tilly, stuffed full of titbits, and about the ingredients of the cakes, stuffed full of E-numbers and hydrogenated vegetable oil. Sally and I had just begun to cotton onto the risks of chemicals in food, but there was no way of explaining this to Molly and I am sorry to say that for the most part we took the easy way out and let her buy and eat whatever she liked. Ironically, Molly had studied E-numbers and chemicals some time before, but only insofar as medications were concerned, and had bought a book detailing the constituents of every medicine under the sun.

Sally or I visited her every day now, administering the pills, clearing and cleaning where we could, and walking the dog, which we really looked forward to. As did Tilly. She went crazy when either of us arrived, leaping up at us, lips curled in canine grin, tail going in frantic gyrations, and her increasingly stout body bent into an increasingly difficult half circle. Then she would gently take hold of our arm in her mouth as the ultimate in her repertoire of loving gestures. We were the recipients of full-on doggy devotion. As soon as the door was open, she would rush out to the car and heave herself onto the back seat, then sit and wait, ears pricked and tail wagging, for however many humans were going to come with her.

If Molly came with us, I enjoyed her company. She loved all pretty shapes and colours, and we would point out Mother Nature's wonders to each other as we walked, but I have to say that this is where Molly stole a march on me. I would spot only the obvious: the bright colours of a late summer flower, a sleepy butterfly meandering by, a pale sun sprinkling the choppy sea with spangles of light. She, however, would see what I didn't.

"Look at all those greens!" she would exclaim, so I would follow the line of her pointing finger. The hedgerow would be full of dark green ivy and its paler flowers, soft hued campion leaves, bright nettles and the mellowness of brambles threaded with purple veins, whilst the ever-wet grass sprouted freshly from the ditch below. All this I would have walked past, not noticing, and it was quite shaming. Sometimes too it would be a particular shape or pattern that caught her eye, and she would exclaim over an unassuming little weed, which you or I would hardly have seen, because its fronds appealed to her. She had always been a naturally arty person, as evidenced by her flower arrangements spread over every surface in the bungalow. But her present mental state seemed actually to increase her awareness of colour and form. I wondered if it was because the absentness of her mind freed it from the cares that occupy you and me on a country walk, and allowed it instead to dwell on the here and now, but it was only when I read a wonderful book by Temple Grandin, called "Animals in Translation", that I discovered the real answer.

Animals? Yes indeed. We are all animals, and let us not forget it! I shall not be able to explain this theory as fully as Temple did, but I will have a bash, and here's how I see it.

Temple is autistic, and the book is written from this viewpoint as much as the animals'. Neither an animal nor an autistic person can be said to have dementia, but, to bring it down to the most simplistic terms, humans have frontal lobes in their brain, which animals do not. These frontal lobes are the first to suffer from any damage e.g., injury, old age, dementia, or a developmental disability such as autism. The more damaged the frontal lobes, the more the brain falls back on its animal level.

One of the many functions of our frontal lobes is to filter the myriad details around us. If they didn't, we would be overwhelmed by these details. And indeed, autistic brains *are* overwhelmed, for they do not have this ability to filter. An example in Temple's book was the boy who got focused on all the screws in the hallway in his school. He had to stop and look at and touch every single one. His frontal lobes were not filtering them out. So, I think that Molly's frontal lobes, although not as badly affected as the young schoolboy's, were incapable of "removing" all the bright displays and plants in her field of vision, and her animal brain took over and made her notice them.

(Another fact that intrigued me was that animals can also hear better than we can - and I am not talking about just a few decibels' difference. What we have always labelled a "sixth sense" in animals - e.g. elephants communicating sub-sonically, cats "knowing" when their owner is coming home - is just better hearing. I, too, have woken from sleep minutes before, say, John coming home from a late meeting, or, years ago, before my parents returned from Cornwall in the night. Was my animal brain hearing the cars before my sleeping frontal lobes did?)

This is just a tiny part of what Temple's book covers, and I would recommend it to anyone interested in brains, animals or both.

On our walks, Molly and I would converse in a desultory fashion. She had never been a great one for long conversations, and most of the chitchat came from me, but we always had much in common, and she was still capable of forming coherent sentences even though she could not always find the word she wanted. Talking of the cottage where she used to live, she was describing some plants to me.

"I had loads of them, all over the ... that field place where I used to put them," she said.

"Do you mean the shrubbery, by any chance, Mother?" I asked wryly.

"Yes, that's it!" she said. Fancy forgetting her shrubbery, the part of her garden she loved the most! Neither of us were worried; we both laughed, and I told her of the television programme about "grumpy old women", one of whom was complaining that she could not remember the word "garden". All she could think of was "squirrel" but she knew that wasn't right, and eventually settled on "that place you go out in". If she was unfazed enough to talk about it on television, what did Molly have to worry about?

There are people, perhaps, who would think our attitude too complacent, that the AD sufferer should be corrected when they use the wrong word, must be made to repeat the right one so that it is drummed into their failing memory. To me, this is no more than mental bullying. Conversing with an AD sufferer may have similarities to chatting with a toddler, but it is not at all the same because with the latter, we are teaching as we talk; the toddler learns as time goes on. An AD sufferer simply forgets, and there is no way they are going to remember, whatever you do. So why not be gentle with them? Don't insist that they put that "broken leg" to the ground and try to walk on it.

So, we carried on laughing *with* Molly at her forgetfulness, and generally enjoying life.

Real life intruded as always, however, and in October we had to make a visit to Dr N who took over from Dr B. Amie, our lovely CPN, was in attendance too. Again I pretended to Molly that we were going shopping and then popping in to the health centre to have her blood pressure checked. This would get us as far as the surgery and, after that, it was up to the doctor. But Molly always behaved herself in front of strangers, and she answered Dr N's "Mini Mental" questions to the best of her decreasing ability. Amie always ran the test past Molly when she visited her at home, but it was some time since I had been in attendance, and it came as a shock to me that day, when Molly did quite badly. Even on the subtracting 7's, which she had always got right, she fell at the second fence.

"What is a hundred minus seven?" asked Dr N.

"Ninety three." She answered confidently.

"What is ninety minus seven?" he continued.

A slight pause, then she ventured, "Ninety."

One more chance. "What is ninety minus seven?"

"Eighty five."

"All right, thank you." No-one ever said anything if Molly got the answers wrong, in the interests of not upsetting the patient, and Dr N moved smoothly on to the next question.

"What is this I am holding?"

"A pen!"

"Can you write a sentence with it?" and he gave her a piece of paper. Once upon a time she would have written something sardonic like "A sentence with it," but this time she just wrote her name.

"Can you read out what you have written?" asked the doctor.

"Molly Pembroke," she replied blithely. Her maiden name.

We struggled on, me sitting speechless - as was required, so no-one noticed. Then the doctor turned to me.

"Your mother is at the point where I should, officially, take her off the Aricept."

My heart plummeted into my boots. I had been dreading that day. Aricept was not a cure, but we were certain that it was helping to keep Molly on a more even keel.

"However, I am not going to do that," ... my heart bounced back to its proper place ... "as it could put her into a steep decline. The time to do it will be when she *has* to go into residential care." Heart wobbled, but stayed put. "Are you coping, or do you have any problems?"

"Well," I said, "we are going along just fine, day to day, except that sometimes she won't take her pills in the morning. But we have had one or two instances of her cancelling planned outings. We make all the arrangements, then she cries off at the last minute, saying she doesn't feel well."

"I think you will have to be more stringent over her taking the tablets. The feeling ill, or that she cannot cope, could be due to a drop in blood pressure. Can you, perhaps, try and monitor this, say, an hour after her taking the pills? Ask her then if she would like to go out."

This dialogue had been taking place in the proverbial how-many-sugars-does-she-take mode, and the doctor and I were both as guilty as each other, but I have to say that, as before, Molly did not seem to mind, or indeed to notice.

I agreed to try his pill monitoring suggestion, and then he did turn to Molly.

"Now, Mrs Smith, do you like living at home?"

"Oh yes."

"Would you like to live in a residential home?"

Good God! I thought. That's cutting straight to the chase! I held my breath to see how she would answer. The question was not such a strange one, but I realised in that split second how conditioned I was to Molly's own mother, our Nan's, reaction to the subject. She would have had complete hysterics at such a question. Nan, crippled with arthritis though she was, had always said she would die rather than spend her last years in a home (I am not sure she realised that that was the actual choice), and that she would prefer crawling around the floor on her hands and knees to being attended by care assistants. Sadly, the fact that we were doing the attending, whilst trying to lead our own hectic lives, had escaped her, and she complained bitterly to her dying day when we finally found it all too much and she did, after all, have to spend her last six months incarcerated in a residential home. But Molly responded quite calmly to Dr N's query.

"Oh no," she replied.

"All right. Who deals with your finances?"

"I do!" she answered confidently.

He knew this couldn't be true, but carried on.

"And who pays the bills?"

"My husband."

I was aghast. Smithy had died twelve years ago. I shook my head at Amie, and said to Molly, "*I* deal with most of it, but you'll just have to take my word!"

"Do you believe that?" asked Dr N of Molly.

"Of course I do!" she replied brusquely. He was just testing her, to see if she understood, but it was nice to see that she did, and also to have her express her confidence in me.

We got up to go, Molly calmly gathering her handbag and coat and smiling serenely at all; me gathering my shattered wits only just in time to ask Dr N about a new drug, Ebixa, that I'd heard about on the radio. He replied that it had been used for years in Germany with no brilliant results, and he would like more information about it before he started using it. So, no hopes there.

That was the last time we visited the doctor. I suppose with so many dementia cases to attend to, he could not keep up personal visits with every one, and obviously reached a point where there was no good reason to keep testing. The patient is on the downward slide, and one day they will have to be put into residential care. Goodbye and next please.

* * * * *

People have often told Sally and me that Molly is lucky to have two daughters to do so much for her. I suppose she is, but we just feel we are doing what comes naturally. After all, would not any son or daughter do the same? Hadn't Molly too been a devoted daughter, and looked after Nan in *her* dotage? Well, yes, but perhaps more in a practical sense than an emotional one.

A little aside here will give you an insight into the complicated creature that is our mother. When she was a little girl, she was devoted to her own mother, Ruby. She would sit on her lap, indulge in heart-warming cuddles, and be totally distraught if deprived of her mother's company. She was equally close, probably even more so, to her father, who doted on his child. When war came, however, and evacuation with it, the fourteen year old Molly was given a choice of location. Because her father was a teacher, she could go with him and his school, and thus remain with her mum and dad. Or she could go with her own school and stay with her friends. She chose her friends.

Nan was devastated. She cried for days and nights, until Grandad told her to stop. "Your duty is to *me*," he chastised her. "Your husband! I want you and need you, but you have a choice. Either go to your daughter, or stay with me. But this grief has to stop." Nan dried her tears, kept her sadness to herself, and plunged herself into Good Works, looking after evacuee children in the village. Family life, as for so many others at that time, was never to be the same again.

When I was seven, Molly's father, my grandfather, died. And Molly stopped believing in God. Her father *was* her god. But she still had feelings for Nan. Putting her arms round her, she said, "You will always have a home with us." Nan told us this, for Molly seldom spoke of anything related to her father's death.

Molly and Smithy were both true to their word, helping Nan and involving her hugely in our family life for years. As those years passed, however, Molly's affection for her mother grew ever less. Nan just seemed to irritate her. Even as children we noticed it, and when we were teenagers Nan would unburden herself to us. "I don't know what I've done to deserve this treatment," she would grieve. It was almost as though Molly resented so much her father dying, that she would rather it had been her mother. She did all the dutiful things, to the day Nan died, but of love there was none. Even Smithy was gentler with Nan than Molly was. Then Molly and Smithy moved to Cornwall, and neither one of them invited Nan to move house and be near them, but just sprang the news on her one day. So, from living ten minutes' walk away, Nan's daughter and son-in-law would now be at a distance of 300 miles. What was more, in later years when Nan made up her own mind to move to Cornwall, after Sally and I did, Molly did her best to try to dissuade her.

Fortunately Nan persisted, and, with her grandchildren to back her, upped sticks at the age of 80 and moved west. Molly objected loud and long, but did join in with the move, shifting furniture, laying carpets, redecorating, being dutiful again. Some years later, when

Nan was very ill, Molly nursed her back to health. But in all the years that I remember, there were no cuddles, no spontaneous laughter, not even any mode of address other than the second person singular, or an occasional "Ruby", Nan's Christian name.

Perhaps Nan had the last word, however. She died in 1994 at the age of ninety seven, but lived on in the depths of her daughter's mind. Eight years later, just after the visit to Dr N, Molly was hearing voices, for she told us, "I don't like all this talk from my mother and her friends."

We did not know that such delusions were a feature of AD, so whereas nowadays we would humour her, Sally tried to explain that Nan had died years before. Of course Molly couldn't remember. She was now finding it increasingly difficult to remember so many things from the past, as well as the present. Not only had she forgotten Smithy's and Nan's demise, but didn't know who Royce's wife was, and had also, we suspected, forgotten Royce as well.

She informed Winnie next door that she had no idea how many children she had.

CHAPTER 11

SHEETS TO THE WIND

Molly was forgetting things on a practical level too, and the house was beginning to lose its pristine order. The carpet needed vacuuming. The ornaments had lost their lustre. The potted plants were un-watered. Even the bath was unused and dusty. The dishes were washed, after a fashion, but the washing up liquid remained redundant in the cupboard under the sink. The washing machine sat ignored in a corner of the kitchen, while dripping items of hand-washed clothes hung for days on an airer in the sherb. Food, however, was still at the forefront of Molly's mind, so the shopping routine at the local Spar continued, albeit with the selection of foods getting increasingly smaller. But at least she could find her way to the village and back, and she was often to be encountered wheeling her trolley basket along the road to and from the village, her large handbag tucked inside.

Like most elderly ladies, Molly was not comfortable without The Handbag, and its whereabouts featured prominently in our own lives. In old-ladylike fashion, she would hide it, and then, when we were all set to go to Spar or out for a coffee, she couldn't find it. I got to know many of the obvious hiding places - cushions, sideboard, top of wardrobe - and it was during a foray into the bedroom, and a rummage through her pile of pillows that I found the bag - and caught a whiff of the bedclothes. "Phew!" I gasped. "I wonder how long since she's changed these sheets?" and pulled them back to look. The bottom sheet was a dull brown colour, woven with dog hairs and covered in the Cornish mud that had dried on Tilly and not brushed off until she went beddy-byes, enticed under the bedclothes by her mum. I hastily covered everything up again while I thought of a ploy. Molly was still firmly independent and would refuse any assistance in doing the washing.

The Smith genes came to the fore. Well, it wasn't the Pembroke ones; they were straight as a die (and if you, like me, have ever wondered what that means, a die is a stamp for marking metal, so it needs to be put on straight). But I remember Smithy's many machinations of old, and I pride myself on having inherited some of his wiliness.

Tilly, as well as putting on weight, had been having some skin problems, partly inherited and partly as a result of her appalling diet. Sally and I knew that Molly fed her handfuls of whatever she herself was eating, usually cake, and we could not even be sure that the dog was still getting normal dog food, so we had taken to feeding that to her ourselves. Tilly now weighed in at about 5 stone, and we would be met with raised eyebrows and tuts every time we took her to the vet, but what could we do? Anyway, the skin problem:

"You know last time we took Tilly to the vet?" I prompted Molly.

"No, not really."

"Well, she's got this skin problem. She does scratch a lot, doesn't she?"

"Yes, she does. I tell her to stop, but she won't."

"Yes, I know. It's very difficult. But," I lied, "the vet did say that it would help if her bed was kept clean."

Silence.

"You do have her in the bed with you, don't you? I know you do, you rascal, so don't try and deny it!" Holding my breath that this approach would work.

"Well, yes, she does get into the bed sometimes."

Sometimes? I didn't have to be a bug on the bed-head to hear, *"Come on, girly, in you get."*

"Well, I think it might be a good idea if we changed the sheets, and I do them in my washing machine. I can get the water a lot hotter than you can by hand, and it will do Tilly good."

"Oh, well I suppose it would be an idea. But I can do it."

"Well, let's go and get the sheets off, shall we?" One stage at a time. Up to bedroom, strip bed, stuff sheets in pillow case, repeat speech about washing machine, agreement reached, we have lift off!

All this might seem a dreadful fuss in order to carry out a simple operation, but if Molly didn't want to do something, we stood two chances of changing her mind; no chance, and a dog's chance. Fortunately the dog got her chance this time, and I repeated the tactics for some weeks. I also got Sally in on the scheme, and we did a brilliant double act, one of us keeping Molly busy downstairs, while the other sneaked upstairs ("Just going to look for your handbag...") and stripped off bedding. In the first two weeks, we got through about ten machine loads of sheets and blankets. Molly had kept piling blankets on, not because it was particularly cold in the bedroom, but because she liked all the different colours. Once everything was washed and dried, we sorted the good stuff from the old and ragged, eventually replacing the whole lot with a duvet ("Isn't this a pretty eiderdown, Molly?"). The old stuff was divided between local charity shops and Clem's dog bed.

Molly's counterpart in America was much more switched on with her laundry, as an email from Adrian demonstrated.

> *Every morning one of the first things Pob does is put a load in the washing machine. We've never quite found out what she washes, and have a sneaky suspicion that most of it doesn't need doing. Still, if it keeps her happy, let her get on with it. But yesterday, although the washing powder is right by the machine, she came into the kitchen, got a bottle of disinfectant*

out from under the sink, and dumped half of it in with the washing. I pointed out the washing powder to her, but she insisted that the disinfectant was what she always used, and that I didn't know what I was talking about. Jill and I suddenly realised that it might be only a small step to Pob's drinking the stuff, so we have now cleared it all out, and I am going to refill the bottles with coloured water, so that everything looks normal. Funny, but this morning she used the washing powder without hesitation.

As the months went by, Molly got used to helping Sally and me strip the bed, and our system seemed to work well. It was a pleasant enough chore, with no complaints or questions from Molly, but she would forget what we had done within minutes and then, when she saw the pillow case bulging with dirty sheets by the back door, she would ask what it was. I would reply, "Oh that's my rubbish," and she would accept this. The good part about Molly's acceptance of our untruths was that it made our lives easier, but the bad part was that it meant Molly was losing more brain cells. But this was inevitable anyway, so we felt we might as well make use of it. Callous again? You bet. But come and try our footwear some time.

Footwear ... stockings ... Christmas. Molly didn't send any cards that year, and didn't ask us any questions about them either (e.g. Had *I* sent them yet?). She forgot many of the people who did still send. Still, I managed to get her to lunch at Carmelin two days before Christmas, and she, John and I had an enjoyable meal together. He was all right with Molly if I was there too, and we managed to make it a merry enough occasion. Afterwards Molly insisted on washing up, which she did perfectly adequately once I had remembered to squirt some w.u. liquid into the bowl, but then she had another of her funny turns, feeling weak, wobbly and peculiar. I had to support her while she tottered the few yards to our spare bedroom, where I tucked her under the duvet and told her to rest. Whatever it was seemed to pass quickly, but I left her there about twenty minutes just in case. Popping my head round the door, I asked, "How do you feel?"

"I feel fine. Just silly."

"You don't need to see a doctor, then?"

"No, I'll be all right."

She did indeed seem to be fine, and she rejoined us for a cup of coffee and some television. A further triumph ensued when I got her to Carmelin for dinner on Christmas Day itself. No dark moods this year, and she enjoyed the day with John and me, having some lunch and exchanging a few little presents. One of these was "From the cats: Fanny, Holly, Jo and Mary" and she asked "Who is Mary?"

"She's our tortoiseshell cat. Here she is! Come here Mary." And Mary obligingly strolled over to be identified and cosseted.

Thirty seconds later, Molly was re-reading the label on the present and she asked again, "Who is Mary?"

"Mary's the cat."

And another thirty seconds, "Who is Mary?" but added surprisingly, "I expect I already asked you." So she did still know how forgetful she was. One thing she had not lost, though, was her love of music, so we turned on the television and spent a relaxing couple of hours watching Swan Lake. We both became lost in the wonderful world of Tchaikovsky's music, the only difference being that I snapped back into the real world and Molly didn't.

"Where am I going to sleep?" she asked in the middle of it, and I had to explain that I would take her home later. Which I did, before it got dark, lit the fire for her, and returned to supper with John. I did have a qualm or two, leaving her there alone, but I knew it was what she preferred, that she was warm and cosy and had her dog. At present, there was nothing more she wanted.

CHAPTER 12

THINGS GET WORSE

A year ago we had encountered the déjà vu syndrome. By 2003, this had faded away and instead we had Molly losing touch with reality. One January day, as Sally was exclaiming over some early snowdrops in Molly's garden, Molly replied vaguely, "Yes, they are nice. Whose garden *is* this?" This was the second time we had witnessed her wondering on the subject. A few days later, I turned up to walk Tilly as usual. "Oh, that's good," said Molly. "I'd been wondering what to do about her. She's not my dog." I left this statement unchallenged, then, indoors, Molly said, "I don't know how long I'll be able to live here."

"Why not?" I asked, puzzled.

"Well, it's not my house."

I had to tell her the truth, even if it confused her. "Yes, it is. You don't need to worry about that. You can stay here as long as you like."

Fortunately this seemed to reassure her. "Can I? Oh good."

It was not all bad. There was a lot that Molly *could* still remember. One important thing at this stage was operating the log burner in the lounge, and it never ceased to amaze us when we saw that she could still do this - probably because it was an everyday occurrence for all the winter months. So each time we encountered a memory blip, we quickly accepted it and focused on the good parts. On the first day of February, however, we were in for a real shock.

Molly had friends, Hazel and Leslie, who lived at Falmouth. She had known Hazel since they were girls living next door to each other, and she remembered both Hazel and Leslie, so one day we arranged to meet for lunch at the Gweek Inn, a few miles away. John and I collected Molly from Parc Bush, where she was eating a cake sandwich (yes, that's right, a piece of cake between two slices of bread), and drove off to the pub to meet Sally and Martin, Hazel and Leslie. We put in our orders, Molly fancying some chips in spite of her recent mini-feast, and all sat down to lunch. We were tucking in with gusto, chatting merrily, when I happened to look across at Molly. She was very quiet, was not touching her food and just didn't seem right somehow.

"Are you OK?" I asked.

"No, not really," she replied, and suddenly all eyes were upon her and a volley of questions fired. Was the food not right? Did she have a headache? Was she hot? Would she like a drink of water? Some fresh air? A definite yes to the latter, and I virtually carried her to Hazel's car, legs buckling - Molly's to start with and mine by the time we reached the car park. Hazel and I got her into the car, tucked her up in a blanket and made her comfortable enough to leave her for a little while. While she sat there and dozed we went back in to finish lunch, but of course the event had put a damper on the occasion. We downed our meals with unseemly haste, said fond and fast farewells and took Molly home. She seemed a little weak and wobbly, but was soon walking about eating cake again. What had been the problem? Was it the heat? Stress? Excitement? Pills? None of these had caused a problem before, so we just didn't know, and there was not much we could do. Except, on a practical level, just one thing, when we got back to Parc Bush. The electrics were playing up again, the bathroom light having discovered how to flip the trip switch, and merrily doing so at every opportunity. Sally and I fiddled about with it until it seemed to be working again, then, erroneously thinking we had fixed everything, said goodbye to Molly and went home.

The next day Molly's wits went AWOL and she went walkabout. A Ruan resident found her two miles from home on the road to The Lizard and phoned Sally who in turn phoned me before driving out to rescue her. Molly had Tilly with her, on a piece of scrap material for a lead, and was carrying a plastic bag stuffed full with cream crackers. She wore her patched gardening anorak, but no hat, and wellies but no socks. It was raining quite heavily and she was wet through.

"Would you like a lift?" asked Sally as she pulled up alongside the unlikely pair. Molly needed no persuasion and climbed in as though everything were perfectly normal. Far from it. I met the carload as they arrived back at Parc Bush and we walked in through the unlocked back door to the living room and a scene of devastation. Not one piece of furniture was in its right place. Chairs had been moved around, cushions were strewn everywhere, the lamp-stand was at a drunken angle against the wall, the television was on the floor and the little television table was lying upside down next to it. Of course the first thought to flash through one's mind was burglary, but it soon flashed out again. It was pretty obvious that Molly had had another turn, perhaps fallen over or thrown a wobbly, or just not known what she was doing for a few minutes. When we divested her of her wet things we found that she was wearing her old grey trousers, tied up with the belt from her plastic raincoat, and no knickers. I fetched her a pair, plus some tights and clean, red trousers.

"You'll feel much better if you change into these," I said.

"Oh thanks," she replied and went off to do so. Half a minute later we found her at the kitchen sink, wearing the knickers over the grey trousers, and the red ones over everything. We tried to persuade her to change, but very soon gave up. It was not, after all, life-threatening. Then we discovered the electrics had tripped off again. Great. But this was not all. For the finale, Sally found a smelly tea towel carefully wrapped round a piece of - brace yourself - poo.

Although we had had experience a-plenty of little doggy accidents throughout our lives, this was our first experience of the poo-wrapping thing. So, although we could easily blame Tilly, why did Molly wrap it up, and in a tea towel of all things? We were mystified. Plus we were not even sure that it *was* Tilly, poor thing. Having walked the dog for two years and more, we knew a Tilly turd when we saw one.

The next day I rang Amie, and she explained that these turns Molly seemed to be suffering were likely to be TIA's (trans-ischaemic accidents occurring in the blood vessels of the brain), and Molly would feel confused and panicked afterwards. She would be calm enough while we were around and she could focus on us, but, when alone, the panic would set in. The TIA's could happen at any time and she would get better after each one, but never to the level she had been before. So life would be a gentle (we hoped) downward slope with occasional drops and occasional smaller rises.

It was helpful to know this. But how much more helpful if we had known in advance. I suppose I should not blame the social services who were, as ever, trying to get several quarts' worth out of a pint pot, and they had indeed furnished us with some quite useful notes. But, since the doctors knew that Molly had, in all probability, had TIA's before, why did they not warn us to expect more, and suggest ways to cope?

Amie did her best, and at this point she offered to arrange a care package for Molly. This would entail someone calling in at Parc Bush at least once a day, and up to three times if needed. What Amie did not tell us, was that this would be a private care package. When she spoke to Sally a few days later and said the package would cost £35-40 per week, Sally had to say a polite "No thank you".

Money can make such a difference in dealing with AD. Back in the USA, Adrian and Jill had a few more pennies than we did, and had succeeded in easing their lives, and enriching Pob's, considerably.

Forgot to tell you this (oh, no!) but we have enrolled Pob in adult day care. The place is about three miles from our home, and looks after old ducks for $45 per day - worth every penny, because Jill and I can get on with our lives without worrying what the old girl is getting up to. It seems a damn good place; the staff are pleasant and very compassionate, and get the old folks doing stuff, playing games, all sorts of things. Pob loves it, calls it her job, and if anyone asks her about her day there she talks about it in exactly those terms - except that she never remembers what they do. Only one small problem - I just hope she isn't thinking of getting a pay cheque at the end of the week! At least she doesn't think that I'm her husband anymore.

This last remark illustrated an interesting difference between Pob and Molly. Although Molly might not remember names, or how many children she had, there seemed to be no confusion over who we were, as long as she saw us on a fairly regular basis. This, of course, excluded my brother Royce. He and Patti worked full time running the inn at Bodinnick, and he had few opportunities to drive the fifty miles to come and see any of us.

At the beginning of March he called round to visit Molly, having not seen her since our wedding the summer before, and she greeted him at the door with "Who are you?" You might expect this from an AD sufferer, but the trouble was, we didn't know if it was genuine amnesia; whether she recognised his face but forgot his name; or if she was merely exercising her sardonic sense of humour.

She forgot this visit of Royce's as soon as he had walked out of the door, and when I mentioned it a few days later she said she could not even remember what he looked like. "Well," I mused, as I went in search of Tilly's lead, "in Royce's case, that's probably just as well!" and her chuckles followed me all the way to the kitchen. When I reached the kitchen table, I did a double-take as I spotted the evidence of Molly's latest trip to the village shops. Her purchases were lined up on the table; all the usual suspects, plus a packet of Ready Brek.

"I didn't know you liked that," I commented, pointing to the alien box.

"Nor did I," she replied. "Who put it there?"

"I don't know. Father Christmas maybe? Do you want to come for a walk?"

"No, thanks. I've only just got in from the shops."

So I took Tilly on my own, coming back some forty minutes later to find Molly looking for her jacket.

"Where are you going?" I asked.

"I want to go shopping, but I can't find my coat." My mouth dropped open like a village idiot's. Surely she had not forgotten her trip of less than an hour before? I shut my mouth, then opened it again, ready to explain gently that she had already been, but was saved from the task when she found the belt to her coat. "Oh," she sighed, "that's no good on its own. I shall have to give up."

"Well, it's pretty horrible out there," I said, hoping she didn't look out of the window and see the sun peeking through the clouds. "I should wait till tomorrow and go then. I'll give you a lift."

Molly agreed to this, so I turned up next day in time to take her to the shops before going on to her doctor's appointment for a general and post TIA check-up - which I had taken care not to reveal to her in advance. We duly set off, did a very small trawl of the Spar shop, just in case she had remembered my promise, then went along to the surgery.

"How are you?" asked the doctor, smiling at her.

"Fine, thank you," replied Molly, naturally.

"Let's just check the blood pressure," he suggested, and proceeded to do so. "Hmm, it is quite high. I think we'd better double the blood pressure tablets, and we'll have a daily aspirin too."

Some doctors are known to prescribe aspirin for anything from in-growing toenails to broken legs, but in this case he was probably quite right to do so. It is well known that aspirin thins the blood, and it is readily doled out to anyone who has had, or is thought likely to have, a stroke. More recent studies have shown that it could well be a cure for all sorts of other things, and I am only surprised that it was not given to Molly much sooner. Maybe it would have prevented the very first TIA's, which caused such damage to the blood vessels that they could well have been the actual cause of Molly's dementia. Maybe a few little aspirins could have prevented the whole sorry story. But maybe that's a surmise too far; no amount of aspirin can cure Alzheimer's. And no matter how many different pills were prescribed for Molly, nothing was going to actually reverse the dementia, and this was forcefully demonstrated by her midnight meandering to Mullion Holiday Park, as mentioned at the beginning of the book, which took place at about this time. Molly's trip was occasioned, we had concluded, by the wretched Parc Bush electrics, which gave a new meaning to trip switch, and we were now determined to get the problem sorted out. Fortunately we knew just the person.

Charlie "I-can-do-that" Goodship was an obliging chap who had recently moved to The Lizard from London, and there was nothing he wouldn't tackle. John and I had added his middle name a few weeks after we got to know him. Although he was qualified only as an electrician, Charlie would take on any job, and we would merely have to show him something broken, or mention a job that needed doing and he would nod and affirm in his sarf London drawl, "Ah c'n do that." This made such a pleasant change from the workman's customary response of sucking of teeth, slow exhalation through puffed cheeks, shake of head, naming of price and then disappearing forever, that we could hardly believe our luck. As it turned out, our luck only lasted two years before Charlie's missus got bored with life on The Lizard, and insisted on moving back to Essex, taking a reluctant Charlie with her. Meanwhile, we made the most of him. He came, he saw, he conquered the electrics, and all was back to normal for a little while at Parc Bush. Did I say normal? We had a bigger problem than the electricity supply. What on earth were we going to do about Molly?

CHAPTER 13

THE PLAN

Although Jill and Adrian's emails often carried a "don't know how much more of this we can stand" flavour, they were obviously prepared for quite a lot more.

> *We have three criteria for deciding to put Pob in a residential home. One is if she loses it mentally to the point where it doesn't matter any more. The second is if she fails physically to the point where she becomes totally helpless. The third is if something like incontinence develops. But we have just added a fourth. It is the point at which we feel that either one of us cannot stand the situation anymore, when we have reached the end of our tether. Gotta be damn careful with that one. Of the two of us, I think Jill will be the first to crack, simply because she is the one who carries most of the load and most of the emotion.*

No-one could argue with the above, but Amie, Sally and I all agreed that it was too soon to think of Molly being put into a care home. She was still fairly independent, had a good quality of life, and was too aware of her surroundings to leave the familiarity of her own abode. For the moment Sally and I didn't bother asking Royce his opinion, assuming that he was too busy running his pub to be of any help in a practical sense. Also, his visits to Molly had become fewer and fewer, since he said he couldn't see the point in driving for an hour and half to visit someone who didn't know who he was and couldn't hold a conversation. One had to agree with him, up to a point, but I think the real problem was that he just couldn't relate to the AD thing, as many people couldn't; including John. I would tell John about What Molly Did and What Molly Did Next, and he found it interesting to hear of, but impossible to handle. He is the most loving, supportive and spiritually mature person I have ever known, but Alzheimer's left him quite helpless. He and Molly had never been big buddies, she being so shy even before the AD, and he, despite all his other attributes, being totally inept at small talk. The fact that Molly was now away with the fairies just served further to estrange them, John finding it impossible to come down to her level and talk about anything at all. He, who could chair any meeting, make speeches off the cuff and expound his views on any subject to a willing (or un-) audience, became totally tongue tied in the Alzheimic presence. If I brought Molly to our house, he would greet her politely, then dive into his office burrow like a frightened rabbit.

In Virginia, Adrian was far less frazzled by the situation and, although Jill bore most of the emotional burden, Adrian did have his uses.

We are still living at Pob's house, he wrote, *and there are all sorts of things that we have to look out for. She puts deodorant in her hair, and hair spray under her arms, and all that shit, and Jill is having to watch her more and more. She has a mania for putting things away, and then it becomes a game of hide-and-seek to try and find what she has done with them. She tidies and "puts" the plastic bags that come from the grocery store, and all newspapers must be folded and stacked neatly. So I play a dirty trick on her. Every day I pull a shitload of them out, unfold them and leave them lying around so that she can do it all again. My reasoning is that while she is doing that she isn't doing anything else that might be a bit more of a problem. Not that she sees it that way. The best one we got from her was, "I don't know what you two would do without me." I think we would have some idea - like move back home for a start.*

All this bore overtones of the tactics we employed with Molly, and another one of the family who seemed well able to cope with her - in fact the only man we knew who could - was Sally's husband, Martin. Molly even allowed him to mow her lawns, and the Parc Bush estate was beginning to look more like its old self, surrounded by neat green swards. Encouraged by Molly's being so at ease with her son in law, Sally and Martin had been debating the situation for some time, and one Sunday morning they phoned to ask if they could come and talk to me and John.

"Of course," I replied. "What's it about?"

"Mother."

"Oh God."

"No, we have a plan, and we'd like to discuss it with you."

They duly arrived, and the four of us sat in the lounge while Sally and Martin told us of Martin's idea. We had already dismissed any possibility of Molly living with either of our households; I knew that Molly's presence would come between John and me, and I was not about to let that happen, and also we had John's sons and grandchildren visiting quite often. I could not risk Molly alarming them as well as her most recently acquired son in law. Sally and Martin's house, at Glebe Place about half a mile from Parc Bush, already had four of them living there, and was too small to squeeze Molly in too.

Most important of all, though, was the fact that the more familiar the surroundings, the better an AD patient can cope with life.

So it would be better to keep Molly at Parc Bush. The mountain, said Martin, must go to Mohammed, and here's how. He and Sally, Wenna and Toana would move out of Glebe Place and into two mobile homes in the garden and paddock at Parc Bush. One caravan would be for Sally and Martin, one for Wenna and Toana. Martin was a fisherman and his catch had been declining over the years, with a corresponding increase in his debts. Therefore, Glebe Place would be let on a long-term basis, which would help with the finances. Molly could stay in her own house and keep her garden which she still loved pottering around in, the Ellises would gain an even bigger garden, and they could keep an eye on Molly for a very large part of the day.

I was astounded. "You are really willing to do that?"

"Yes," confirmed Sally. "We'll look after Molly for as long as we can cope, and put off the evil moment of putting her in a home. We think it's a great idea."

"Well, so do I, if *you* do it, because I have to say I would never dream of doing that myself, nor having Molly here. If you are happy, I am willing to go along with it."

So was John. And the girls, after initial objections and face-pullings, were coming round to the idea of living in a caravan. So, why not? We set the wheels in motion, as it were. The first step, however, was to get it past the local district planning office. There was a distinct possibility that someone might find a cure for AD first.

* * * * *

To be fair to Royce, I have to give him a mention here. When I phoned to tell him of our plan, he was quite agreeable to it, but astounded me by saying that, if it didn't work, he and Patti were prepared to have Molly. It had actually been Patti's idea. "I would have expected you to help me look after *my* parents if necessary," she said. There was no answer to this, and Royce wisely kept quiet, although he might just have sent up a silent prayer of thanks that Patti's expectations had never had to be put to the test, her own parents having gone to their reward some time back. "So," she continued, "I am prepared to help look after *your* mother."

"Well," I told him, "that is sweet of Patti, but the main purpose, for the moment, is to keep Molly in her own home, and this is the only way we can do it. If it doesn't work out, we'll come back to you!"

And with this threat looming over him, Royce - like me - prepared to give the Ellis scheme his whole-hearted support. Having applied to the council for permission to site the caravans, I now wrote to Molly's GP and to Amie to gain their written support for the project. We knew all this would take some months, but it was only March and we hoped things would start happening by late summer. Meanwhile Molly continued taking her regular exercise. In early April, only three days too late for All Fools Day, she arrived at the house next door to

Winnie and Albert at 11 pm. We don't know why. She had apparently got out of bed and thrown on the first things she could find, for she was dressed, after a fashion, but had stopped short of putting any shoes on, then headed out. Fortunately Ruan Minor is the sort of village where everyone knows who is doing what, where, when and to whom, and the good neighbour knew, it being Friday, that Sally and Martin were at the pub. She rang Cadgwith Inn and delivered her glad tidings. Wenna, who seldom drinks alcohol, was with her parents, so was able to drive her mother safely back to Ruan Minor. Sally, however, had indulged in several Liebfraumilches, and although she told us that she had to take Molly's arm to lead her home, it was more likely a case of the blind (drunk) leading the blind. This good neighbour often kept an eye on Molly, and if she saw her go from the village direction towards Parc Bush, she would go outside and check to make sure Molly turned into Parc Bush gateway and didn't continue up the road. Molly was lucky to have such kind people so near to her.

As soon as Sally told me about Molly's latest adventure, I rang Amie to ask her advice; then rather wished I hadn't. Amie listened carefully and said that if it got really bad or dangerous, Molly could be sectioned. I was not familiar with this term.

"What do you mean?" I asked.

"Sectioned under the Mental Health Act," explained Amie, "following Section Three which means she'd have to be put in a Home."

Keeryst! My mother *sectioned*? No way!

"But," continued sweet Amie, "Molly manages very well considering that she is severely mentally impaired. So I don't think it should come to that yet."

Severely mentally impaired? My mother? Yes, Jane, your mother. Get real. What a shock it was to register those words and recognise the truth that had been waving its arms at us, and shouting *Hello?* for years.

And yet ... soon after that, on a bright and breezy day in April, Molly came to lunch and a walk with a crowd of us, and everyone was *so* impressed with her. Not only was she physically fit, but she was able to maintain bursts of chatty conversation with several different people. She even remembered the event long enough to say afterwards that she really enjoyed being with friends, which of course she always had, and which made me feel guilty for not arranging such things more often.

The next day, I drove her to Spar for a few groceries. As I had just thrown the bag of laundry onto the back seat, she climbed in after it, and then asked when we got to the shops if I needed it with me. Although she was not so daft as to think I needed to take dirty sheets with me round the supermarket, she had forgotten within the space of three minutes what the bag contained. It dawned on me that this was another instance of her need for reassurance. She had recently begun to ask constant questions about what she should do: where to sit in the car, whether to put the pillowcase on the pillow, was she to put her coat on, should she come with me? Fortunately my responses seemed to keep her happy, and she was quite biddable. One day when we called at the jewellers in town to collect my mended watch she stood quietly waiting and told the assistant sunnily, "I just do what I am told."

"Well," I said, "there's a first time for everything."

And so we laughed again. But, sadly, Amie was right. Molly *was* severely mentally impaired. Alzheimer's is such a strange disease. Notorious for causing loss of memory, its effects go far deeper. Molly, who had always buzzed to and from the shops, but few places else, was now enthusiastically making up for lost time. We wondered whether we should rename her Mole, as she would pop up unexpectedly all over the place. A report from Sally's friend Sarah described a visit to some people in Cadgwith, complete strangers to Molly. They answered a knock on the door, to be greeted by Molly saying, "Hello! I've come for my usual things!"

Although utterly mystified, they didn't like to turn her away, so invited her in, and fed her a banana and some chocolate biscuits.

"Thank you very much," said Molly, polite as ever, after she had finished the mini fest. "How much do I owe you?"

"No, no, that's quite all right," they demurred.

"Oh, well thank you again. I had better be off then." And off she toddled, arriving back home quite safely. We would not even have heard of this voyage had these good people not mentioned it to Sarah and asked her if there were any new age travellers around. Obviously Molly was once again dressed to kill! Sarah knew of "Sally's Mum" and guessed correctly that it was her.

The next rescue mission was carried out when friends of ours, who live near the church in Ruan, looked out of their window and saw Molly wandering around their courtyard. They too knew of Sally's Mum, so rang Sally and then very kindly walked Molly home.

Thank goodness for our wonderful circle of friends. Not three days later, Anna drove past Molly along the busy road that joins up with the Lizard-Helston road, recognised her as she passed, jammed on the brakes and went back to her. "Like a lift, Molly?"

"Oh, thank you, that would be nice," and in she got. Molly was getting enough free rides to put an entire fleet of taxis out of business. Anna took her to Sally's, and Sally took her home. When they got to Parc Bush, Molly got out of the car, looked around and said, "I recognise this."

"Yes," said Sally, ever one for the brutal truth. "You live here."

Molly giggled. And so did anyone else to whom we related these tales. But one person we did not tell was Amie. We did not want Dr N sectioning her just yet. Besides being, in our opinion, unnecessary, it made her sound like a piece of pie.

It was all very well laughing, but we really needed to expedite The Plan before Molly did something really silly or dangerous. So Sally rang Kerrier Council who were being incredibly dilatory. Nothing new there, then.

"I am sorry for the delay, but we must do things by the book," intoned the officer in charge.

"That's all very well," responded Sally crisply, "but Mother is *not* doing things by the book."

"Ah, yes. I see what you mean. Well then, go ahead with your caravan plan and please keep me informed of your mother's meanderings."

Why? Was he short on laughs?

CHAPTER 14

MORE WALKABOUTS

While Sally was engaged with most of the practical work on this caravan project, I tried to do my bit. Firstly, in case of more walkabouts, I took a picture of Molly and Tilly, did a write up entitled "Have You Seen This Lady?" and distributed the notices all round the village, plus one to Helston police station. Then, as it was time to tell Molly of our plans, I engaged her in a gentle chat while we ate strawberries in her sherb one warm July day. It was not an easy subject to wade into, as we were not at all sure how she would react to a gypsy encampment in her garden, but I stuck a toe in the water and started with, "Do you remember visiting Barbara down the road yesterday?"

"No. Who's Barbara?"

"She's a friend of mine who lives about half a mile away. I think you got lost and she brought you home. Another strawberry? Go away, Tilly, you won't like them."

"Oh, that was nice of her. Yes please."

"They're rather yummy, aren't they? Mmmm. Actually, I think you've got lost a couple of times lately, and we're a bit worried about you."

"Oh, I didn't know I was that barmy!"

"No, you're not barmy, just a bit absent minded. It does tend to happen as you get older. We're all getting forgetful these days, aren't we?"

"Don't know. Can't remember!" she cackled.

"Yeah, right. Anyway, short of locking you in ..." more chuckles ... "what do you think we should do about it? Here you are, have the last one. *No*, Tilly, go and lie down."

"Thanks. I don't know."

"Well," I said, licking my fingers and wiping them on the dog. "How about a note on the gate telling you not to go out?"

"Yes, you could do that, I suppose."

"It would mean you not going out on your own."

"Oh dear."

"But that won't really matter. Sally and I can shop for you, take you into town or wherever..."

"Oh good! Let's go now!"

"OK, in a while ... and you can still walk Tilly in the garden."

"Yes, I suppose so."

"Well, we'll try it. But you know you won't remember this conversation."

"Probably not. Have we got any cake?" Tilly leapt up again and reapplied her Hopeful face. I never did get round to discussing the caravans.

The next day John and I put up two "Don't go out" notices on the gates, screwing them on really firmly with the biggest screws we could find. Tentatively we let Molly view them when she came to wave us goodbye.

"What are *they* doing there?" asked Molly. "They are very strange." Too strange to be allowed to stay. Within two days she had applied determination and a giant screwdriver, and the notices vanished. The walkabouts continued.

* * * * *

In the middle of that summer, we had a surprise visit from yet more old friends of Molly and Smithy. Half a dozen ex-members of the skin-diving club had rented a self-catering cottage for a week and were revisiting all their old diving-holiday haunts. Not all of these good people were from up country; two of them, Dudley and Norma, lived a few miles from us at St Martin-in-Meneage, and we were in fairly regular contact with them. Dudley was a builder, and had done lots of work for several members of the Smith family, whilst Norma and Molly had been good pals up until a few years ago. So, what had happened since? Norma's mother, Mavis, that's what. She too had the dreaded AD, and although Norma and Dudley were happy to have her living with them, and coped tremendously well, Mavis took up a lot of their time. Although we were not in touch regularly, I would occasionally bump into them in town and hear the latest tales: Mavis tearing pieces of toilet paper off the roll, folding them up and sticking them behind the bathroom mirror; looking in the mirror asking Who is that lady? throwing her lunch across the table; and the scariest, Mavis making an appearance wearing nothing but her cardigan with its sleeves up her legs, and her knickers on her head. Yes, of course we laughed. And, what is worse, could not begin to imagine that Molly would ever reach that dotty state.

Now we all met again (without Mavis) at the Cellars restaurant in Cadgwith. Even Royce had come along from Bodinnick on his motorbike. Molly did not join in the conversation, but was happy to sit and listen as always. I don't think she recognised anyone except Norma and Dudley, but everyone made a great fuss of her, and one of the lads, Malcolm, gave her a big hug and reminded her about their Thursday evening visits to Crystal Palace Sports Centre to swim, when Malcolm would drive Smithy's car with Molly as passenger. I think that Adrian was not the only one to be impressed in those bygone days by the contents of Mother's bikini.

The tea and conversation flowed delightfully, the air full of laughter and do-you-remembers, but eventually I found myself beside Norma and the conversation came round to Mavis.

"So, how is your mother?" I asked.

"She's all right," replied Norma, "but we've got her in a home now."

"What, permanently?"

"Oh yes. It's a lovely place, The Gables at Redruth. She's been going there for day visits for ages, but we just can't cope any more at home, so we moved her in last month."

"So she's happy there, is she?"

"Oh yes. The staff are lovely, and they're used to dementia patients. Just as well." Norma pulled a wry face. "We had such a time with her at nights. She would get up at all hours and wander around, take off her nappy..." (*nappy????* *No, no.* *Not our Molly...*) "...and hang it round her neck. Then she would fill the bath, but could only reach the hot tap. We woke up one night and heard her yelps of distress - she was trying to climb into the boiling hot water. So we hid the plug. But next time she stuffed a towel down the plughole. We had to turn off the water at the mains each night."

"Oh, my God ..." but there was more.

"She'd take off her nappy at every opportunity ..."

"Wet or dry?" I heard myself ask. Did I really want to know?

"Well, wet, because it was uncomfortable."

"So I suppose it made sense to her to remove it."

"Yes, but then she'd hide it in a drawer, or under the mattress, or at the bottom of the wardrobe. We had to play Hunt the Nappy every day, and we could usually sniff it out, even if we couldn't see it!" and Norma laughed aloud.

"Christ ..." but she hadn't finished.

"She *could* get to the bathroom, but to make it easier for her we had a commode in her room too. But she used to take out the potty bit and sit on the commode without it to do a jobbie. So we put a piece of plastic and a towel on the floor under it."

"Did that do the trick?"

"No, she hid them both and did another jobbie."

"Jeez ... well." Words were failing me. "So now she's in the ... home. Do you get to see her very often? Does she recognise you?"

"Oh, yes, we visit her. If she's been sleeping, and wakes up and sees me, she says, "Oh it's you." But if I go in and she's already awake, all I get is a blank stare. And if she does decide to talk, she leans forward, as though she's going to tell you a secret, then says, "What I say is ..." and that's it."

By now, folks were standing to go, and that was the last I got to talk to anyone else that afternoon, but by then I was so depressed that I didn't really want to. It was all quite awful. I felt sorry for

Norma for having to make that decision, and for Mavis at having to endure Alzheimer's. But mostly for Wenna, who had made the mistake of joining our table and sitting opposite us. I don't think she had come to tea with the idea of learning how to cope with adult nappies and other demented doings.

During the next few days I did some serious soul-searching. All the horrible stuff that Norma had told me about her mother suddenly sank in and I thought, "Is that really what awaits my own mother? Please God, no!" I related it all by e-mail to Adrian, and concluded with ...

"I do sincerely hope that the good Lord, whoever and wherever he is, sees fit to take her before all that. I am not ashamed to admit that hope, and have no doubt at all that most other offspring would wish the same for their aged ones, and for themselves".

Adrian's reply was immediate:

> *Regardless that you say, quite rightly, that you are not ashamed, let me give you the benefit of my experience. There is nothing evil or wicked in your thoughts re Molly, and nothing wrong with wishing for her early demise. All of this is completely normal, and does not make you any less moral, or caring, than anyone else. As a matter of fact, after a conversation with the heart specialist at the hospital, Jill nixed the idea of a pacemaker for Pob, and also installed Code Blue - do not resuscitate.*
>
> *All of the above comes down to the reasons why we try so hard to keep Pob happy, difficult as it is sometimes. Someone you love slipping away, day by day, is a helluva lot worse than death, pure and simple, over and done with. I see Jill handling it all very bravely, and competently, but I wonder how much is being bottled up.*

* * * * *

During the next few months, most of the walkabout rescue operations were carried out by Sally and pals, but John and I received a phone call one September evening from dear old Wally about half a mile up the road from Parc Bush. Wally, who was not in good health, would spend hours just sitting by the window watching the world go by. He recognised Molly from his "Have You Seen..." notice and called me immediately. "She and the dog are heading for the Mullion road," he said.

This was the busy main road along which Molly had marched on the night of her holiday park outing. I ran to the garage, backed out the car, John leapt in beside me, and we did 0 to 50 mph in three minutes. It would have been faster, but it is not possible to get out of second gear up our bumpy lane. We reached the Ruan turning to find

Molly only yards from the main road, wheeling her trolley basket, with Tilly plodding along beside her without a lead. This was beyond funny. We screeched to a halt, thanking God and Wally that we'd caught Molly in time. However, all signs of panic had to disappear before we approached her, or she would become agitated, so I got out of the car and strolled over to her.

"Hello! Fancy seeing you here? Would you like a lift?"

And in she got once more, followed by Tilly and trolley. I peered inside the basket. It contained a pair of wellies, a pair of shoes, one coat and a tin of cotton reels.

The next day I bought Tilly a reflective collar and lead, in case Molly and her mutt went on a midnight meander. Then I got in touch with Charlie, our electrician friend, and asked him if he could put up some very big, i.e. non scaleable, panels on the gates at Parc Bush, and a bolt on the outside. "Yeah, Ah c'n do that, " he replied as always, and he did. Once this was done, it effectively meant that Molly was now locked into her grounds. Tough measures, but these were tough times.

Sally and Martin were now working on clearing the ground in Molly's garden and paddock so that they could move the caravans in. Still unsure of Molly's possible reaction to our plan, I became my father's daughter once more and embroidered the truth. Suggesting a little amble down the garden, I took her to where the caravans would be and made my opening gambit.

"Sally and Martin have great problems, did you know?"

"No, what's the matter?"

"They owe so much money, because Martin's fishing has been so bad, that they have got to move out of their house and let it. So they'll have nowhere to live. We thought if they moved in here, in a little caravan, it would help them, and be company for you."

This appeal to Molly's helpful nature did the trick. "Yes, I suppose it would," she nodded, and I gave a sigh of relief. As time went on, Molly actually became quite keen on the idea and would happily wield spade, pick and shovel whenever Sally and Martin turned up to work. I am not sure that she remembered why they were doing all this, but she had always enjoyed team-work and family projects, so this became just one more. Sometimes it even became difficult to prise her away so that she could come and help me with the shopping. But we continued with the Tesco run, her special favourite. She really liked strolling along pushing the trolley and peering at everything, expressing a particular delight at all the coloured displays on the shelves. Like the flowers and hedgerows, it was probably a frontal lobe thing, but nevertheless this aspect of the supermarket slog is actually something we all miss while charging around trying to get the shopping shopped in double quick time and get home again.

How I would have loved to slow down. Or even to have time to think about doing so. School work was becoming ever more manic and I was at my wits' end trying to fit in those four mornings each week, plus running our home and large garden, and visiting Molly four days a week. She was having more fun in her AD mode than I was in my normal one.

*   *   *   *   *

Although I was weary, I was seldom weary of Molly herself, and enjoyed her company as I had done all my life. Across the pond, however, it was a different story.

> *Last night Jill and I put our cards on the table concerning our feelings of resentment towards Pob. Jill, strange though it seems, actually resents her more than I do, but this is mainly because she is Pob's daughter and Pob stays closer to her. If I am in the kitchen, for example, cooking or washing up, Pob keeps away from me, probably because I am a man and "mustn't be bothered". But Jill has only to try and make herself a drink, or a sandwich, and Pob is right there with her, trying to help. This gets on Jill's nerves so much she wants to scream at her, but that would be futile. So we have agreed that, where possible, I will carry more of the load, allowing Jill the occasional escape. Of course, when it is me who is Pob-sitting, she asks me every five minutes, Where is Jill? All this is not going to last for ever. But be prepared for this resentment thing, and don't feel guilty about it when it happens.*

After reading this, I almost felt guilty because I *didn't* experience any resentment. Obviously, I did not have Molly living with me as Jill and Adrian had Pob, and this was a crucial difference. However, I did get to see how they might be feeling when, a few weeks later, I had Molly at Carmelin for a few hours. In former days, we could have gone for a walk, sat reading or doing crosswords, but now she either would not or could not do those things. As it was a rare afternoon off, I wanted to flop and read the paper, but she couldn't seem to settle, had already perused the photo album six times, and didn't want to read anything else. I realised that she could not actually follow the plot of a book or even a magazine article. So, sad and guilty, I took her home earlier than planned. It occurred to me that I had no idea what she would do at home. Once upon a time she would spend her days in the garden and her evenings indoors, either sewing, knitting (which she could do while watching television), typing letters, doing crosswords or reading books. Now she could no longer do any of this, so how did she fill her day? What did she like to do, apart from looking at photos and eating cake? And she couldn't do either of those for hours on end, could she?

Pob's kitchen keenness was, I think, a girl-thing of wanting to help. It came from generations of having to do just that, and it was not easy to let go. I wondered; when does the dividing line appear? When do we stop being useful and become a pain in the bottom? Kitchen-wise, Molly always wanted to help too, and if she had been with us for a meal, she would head for the washing up at the speed of light. The trouble was, she forgot (a) that we had a dishwasher, and (b) to use any washing-up liquid, so the dishes really only got rinsed. If there were just a few, I could leave her to get on with it, and load them into the dishwasher later. If there were a lot, I would gently lead her in another direction.

(Pob, according to Jill, used the same soapless tactics, and when questioned, replied that it was harmful to hands, pointing out, as evidence, the writing on the bottle that said, "Tough on grease, gentle on hands." Jill gave up!)

Our best solution was to find Molly something to do, even though, like having a child to help, you can do it quicker yourself. One could come unstuck even here, like an old friend of Molly's whose husband also had AD. When asked by his wife to fetch two wineglasses, he came back with a hot water bottle.

Sometimes Molly or Pob could not find things because they had forgotten where they were; usually because they had put them somewhere odd. But in other cases, they did find what they were looking for. At least, they *thought* so.

An e-mail from Adrian put it very well.

It is not a universally known fact that Jill likes a teaspoonful of whisky in her tea. When she came home from work yesterday, and had her usual cup of tea with Pob, she couldn't find her bottle of whisky, because it had been "put away". But Pob said she knew where it was, and went to the dining room sideboard. Fair enough so far because there is booze in there too, but she came back with a box of coins, loose change, picked out a dime, and said, "Here it is, will this do?" Jill was so gob-smacked that she couldn't answer, so Pob repeated, "Here is your whisky. Shall I put it in your tea?"

As for Pob's own cup of tea, I usually make it for her. But one day last week she said that she would do it. As she has been making tea for about ninety years, it is reasonable to assume that she has the hang of it, but I had a twinge of doubt, so I slunk out to the kitchen to spy on her.

She picked up the kettle to tip the water into the pot, but was unable to hold and aim the water properly, and it was going all around the teapot as well as in it. Worse, she was holding the teapot with her other hand, not by the handle, but with her hand around the top of the pot. She sloshed boiling water everywhere, and it was only by a miracle that none of it touched her hand. She had no idea that the water would have scalded her, or that that there was anything unusual in what she was doing. We look upon the making of a cup of tea as so simple that I just could not imagine her being unable to do it, and never realised how dangerous it could be. But she has now made her last cuppa. We really do have to try to stay one step ahead.

The perceived wisdom is that, to keep an AD patient occupied, a long repetitive task was always best, but that ruled out simple stuff like for pouring a drink or making one sandwich. Sadly, however many they made, Molly and Pob would always be at least one sandwich short of a picnic.

CHAPTER 15

TURNING UP THE HEAT

One day during the school summer holidays I had popped into Tesco's, on my own for once, but met a friend from school at the veggie counter. Although we did not see much of each other in the classroom or office, we were on the same wavelength and often shared a laugh or a problem. She now asked me how had my summer been, and I realised, as I answered her, that it had been exhausting. Living at Carmelin and having the chalet to let was like running two houses; the summer was the time when all the painting, pressure washing, outdoor repairs, gardening, etc was done, and although John and I shared the tasks, they did represent a whole lot of work, especially bearing in mind that we were not exactly spring chickens. Added to this, we had had endless friends and family visiting throughout August, and, pleasant though that was, I had had no real break. I dreaded the thought of going back to school the first week of September, whilst having to keep up with my daughterly duties.

"I don't think I can hack it any more," I sighed, and then, hardly believing what I heard myself add, "something's got to give, and I think it might be school."

I had been working at school for six years now, and had the job more or less at my fingertips. It was a job that many mothers coveted; so handy, they thought, for fitting in with the children's own hours. If only it were that simple; and, in the good old days, it was. If you could handle a typewriter and tend to a grazed knee, the job was yours. These days, thanks to a government ever more eager to prove their "worth", much of the secretary's load was taken up with computer statistics. That was bad enough, but worse was the fact that they kept moving the goalposts. Secretaries nationwide had to keep running to stand still; the county councils could not handle all the training and retraining courses needed; the county helpline had a permanent waiting list; and the result was an overworked, demoralised, debilitated workforce. It wasn't much better for the teachers, but that's another story. Some secretaries booked early retirement, some booked a place in therapy, others threw tantrums. I did the latter often, with the result that, far from earning anyone's sympathy, most of the staff avoided me.

That is the nutshell version. Back at home I did some speedy Can I Leave School? calculations and decided that yes, actually, I could. John, fully supportive as always, encouraged me, so, on the first day of the autumn term, I took my carefully written notice with me, waited until I was alone with our Headteacher, and took a deep breath.

"I need to talk to you, Anne," I said.

"All right," she said, with her usual sunny smile. "Go ahead."

"I have to go."

"Go where?" she asked, looking somewhat bewildered.

"Go ... leave ... hand in my notice. I can't do this any more!"

"Oh no!" she said, "You can't mean it! I will feel I am losing a friend." And tears sprang to her eyes. I was astounded. I had expected her to be maybe a little surprised, but I had never encountered that reaction when I left any other job. We discussed the matter, and later I spoke with Pauline, my job-share partner. Pauline was eager to do more hours, and although I warned her of the pitfalls, she was quietly insistent that she could do it, so, after I had confirmed her as certifiably insane, we finally settled on the most simple solution, viz., a job swap. Pauline would do my four days and I would do her one. We would run a trial for two terms, starting after Christmas, and if the "sec's change" didn't work, we would think again. I looked forward to a less frenetic life later in the winter.

The season brought other problems at Parc Bush. Although Molly still remembered *how* to operate the woodburning stove, she now often forgot to actually *do* it. Sally and I had to add it to our daily job list, and would carry a box of matches and kindling with us, because Molly either tidied them away, so that we wasted time searching, or the matches, having been kept in the dank atmosphere of an unheated Parc Bush, would sullenly refuse to emit so much as a spark. One of us would light the fire each afternoon after walking Tilly, hoping that Molly would remember to keep it going. We were not at all sure that she would, but, since we *were* sure that she went to bed as soon as she got cold, and took her dog-hot-bottle with her, hypothermia would not be a danger.

However, even if the lounge and the bed were warm for part of the time, the rest of the house was like a tomb. It was time to get in touch with Charlie again. Could he install some night storage heaters?

"Yeah, Ah c'n ... &c' " and he did. Not only that, but we trusted him enough to tell him the whole story, and confess that Molly would not approve of our efforts to increase her comfort. She had always hated central heating, dismissing it as "horrible and stuffy" so we had to employ subterfuge like never before. We had the heaters delivered to Sally and Martin's address, and Martin brought them to Parc Bush piecemeal while Molly was out. We were optimistic that, once the heaters were installed, she would not remember that they hadn't been there all along. Charlie's initial presence was explained away with a fictitious electrical fault, and then we arranged several trips out for her.

"We'll keep her out of the house as much as we can while you're here, Charlie," I explained. "But this does mean you'll have to make your own coffee. Is that all right?"

"Yeah, thass all right. Milk in the fridge, is it?"

"Yes, next to the saucepans and dog biscuits!"

"Righto." Nothing fazed our Charlie. And so, bless him, he became a fellow conspirator. This worked brilliantly. Except for one day when he turned up unexpectedly and Molly was there on her own. We had had no chance to take her away, as it were. Luckily she behaved herself and left Charlie to get on with fixing the "fault".

"I don't remember anything wrong," she protested mildly.

"Well, yer wouldn't, would yer?" responded Charlie cheerfully, which seemed to satisfy her. Revenge, however, was a dish best eaten cold, and the next day Charlie greeted me at the gate with, "She's 'ad me cable!"

An entire roll of electric flex had been disappeared as only Molly knew how. Search as we might, it was not to be seen, and it never did surface - and we are talking, here, about something as big as a small cartwheel. Charlie had to go and buy another one. We found a few other oddities during our searches though; an arrangement of flower heads and banana slices on a plate in her bedroom; a photograph album with most of the pages torn out at the back of a kitchen cupboard; a stack of neatly rolled up empty crisp packets in the bathroom cupboard; and her duvet, complete with cover, folded carefully and placed on the chest under the window in the downstairs study. She would never have found it when she needed it. So that was another check to add to our daily list, along with pills, dog walk, food and lighting fire. Then I discovered that she had unplugged the freezer. Fortunately the food was still frozen, and she did a good job of mopping up and cleaning out while I walked Tilly. We then put all the food back, plugged the freezer in again, and I put a "do not remove" notice on the plug.

Charlie finished his job, and the heaters were switched on. After a few days I even risked telling Molly all about them and, amazingly, she agreed it was a good idea. But she then forgot this and for a week she went round religiously switching off every single heater. Each day Sally or I had to switch back those that had been turned off, and even when we put the strongest parcel tape over the switches Molly still managed to work them through the tape. We hung on grimly, and eventually the novelty wore off for Molly and she left them alone. She had other distractions to engage her.

In early December the caravans were at last moved into the field. Molly was very interested in all this at first, poking around and "helping" Sally. Then one day she completely forgot what was going on and became confused and cross. I came along later that day and took her on a tour of the caravans all over again, explaining what they was all about, and repeating the reasons why Sally and Martin were going to live here. For good measure I added, "And it will be good to have someone around for when you get even more old and decrepit." She laughed, as I knew she would, and I believe she was relieved, for a few seconds of memory span, to know that there would be company for her in the future. Soon Christmas was upon us, and we enjoyed further triumphs with her helping me to festoon the tree at Carmelin, and then getting her here two or three times over the holidays, including lunch on the day, with Angus and Hamish, followed by prezzies all round. I gave her all sorts of little things that I had individually wrapped over the last week, and at the last minute I found a pair of new mittens that I'd had given to me and didn't need. I was so fed up with wrapping by then, that I got her to gift wrap the gloves herself. This not only saved me a task, but gave her something to keep her busy, which she enjoys, and of course by the time she opened them she had forgotten all about them. Hamish thought this was really funny, and I explained it was the laugh-don't-cry approach. The gloves were really for children, and gaily showed all sorts of different balls - football, rugby, cricket, etc - and she peered at them and asked, "What are all these things?"

"Balls" I said.

"Same to you, with knobs on!" she replied. It never failed to stun me when she came out with things like this; from a memory that was all but defunct, she could still, on occasion, find something that entirely fitted the moment.

Following presents, we all watched Stuart Little on the television, and Molly enjoyed it so much that I let the visit go on longer than I had planned, and drove her home in the dark. This was not good, as she became disorientated, and endless questions followed. Even on a daily basis this could include:

- Are you coming back?
- Why don't they do something about this mess? (Muddy lane, autumn leaves, puddles, anything that wasn't tidy).
- How far is it?
- What are we doing now?
- And you're going to....?
- And I'm going to...?
- Who's Tilly?
- How far is it now?

And now, at night, these were repeated ever more often. She had, however, apparently remembered her afternoon out, in a vague sort of way.

"I used to do ... these things..." she mused, "but now..." and tailed off. But I knew exactly what she meant. "I used to go to parties at Christmas and have lots of fun, but now I don't know what's going on and I get confused, so I stay at home till someone fetches me." Although she was often fairly lucid, the later it was in the day the more confused and lost for words she got. In order to work out what she meant, one had to apply the present situation and surroundings, the last action or subject of conversation and her likely thought processes. If in doubt, a non-committal or concurring answer would usually do, or, if in real doubt, I would ask her what she meant, but I did try to avoid that!

The next day, a beach walk brought forth the following puzzle.

"Is it all right for them" (pointing at the dogs) "to leave their little things?" Molly's hand actions mimed a small thing about the size of a poop, so I asked if she meant dog mess.

"No, not mess, but ... the story of it all."

I failed completely on this one. She could see I was flummoxed so she said fairly quickly that she didn't suppose it mattered, and I agreed. Nowadays I would not even try to interpret, but would calm her by assuring her that, yes, it was quite all right for the dogs to ... leave their little things. Call my method deceitful or patronising, and you might be right; but Molly has never questioned my "understanding" of her speech. Even all those years ago, she did not seem to know if she was using the wrong word, provided I went along with it, and the less I questioned her, the more relaxed she was. So we had entire conversations where I was only vaguely aware of the subject, and these days, when this has progressed often to talking complete gibberish (she, not me - not yet!), we still manage to have our little chats. I would recommend this method for anyone dealing with a dementia patient, but I hope that most carers have already discovered it for themselves.

Although, to our knowledge, there was no history of dementia in our family, we had had a little practice at odd conversations with Nan. She lived to 97 and had gone a little potty in the last few months, but at that age perhaps she was entitled to. Because of failing physical health, she had spent these months in a residential home just a few miles from her own house, so maybe it was only natural that she thought, for example, that the home's resident cat was hers. "She followed me all the way here!" she would boast. Sally's reply of "She's not your cat, Nan. Jane is looking after *her*, this is the Home's cat," would leave Nan looking confused and disappointed, so what was the point of contradicting her? When Nan told me of the cat's incredible journey, I would, out of some kind of instinct, merely say "Really, Nan? Gosh, how clever of her!" By the time Molly was starting to say strange things, we learned very quickly to humour her in a similar way. This is apparently known as the

Habilitation Approach, although I did not learn this term until years later. But we all had so much to learn in the years ahead.

The main thing now was that Molly seemed bright and chirpy for much of the time. I believe she had gone through the stage of realising that something was wrong, with the accompanying anxiety and depression, and had come out the other side, accepting life as it was, and learning to rely totally on us for direction. However, I was also acutely aware that she had anxious moments when alone, and once or twice, when I had been about to leave after walking Tilly, she asked me, "Must you go? I do hate being alone." This was the hardest thing to deal with, and never failed to bring a lump to my throat. We spent so much time being brave, bolstering her as well as ourselves, and burying our heads in the sand re much of the future, but that sort of unexpected event had the power to knock me sideways. So I soon changed my leave-taking tactics, and avoided any immediate distress by saying, "I'm just nipping home to put the washing out, then I'll be back."

"All right," she would say chirpily. "How long will you be?"

"Oh, about twenty minutes."

"OK! See you in a minute then."

She would wave me off, before going back indoors quite happily and forgetting I had even been there, and I would go home and stay there.

Obviously, I knew that she did get anxious when left alone, and so I looked forward fervently to having Sally and Martin living on site. Not only would it give Molly much needed company, but it would also remove our ever-present worry of wondering if she was safe, secure and happy. The Ellises' house move, together with my giving up most of my school hours and having more time to devote to Molly, should mean more quality time for us with her. At the end of 2003, Molly's seventh year into Alzheimer's (7AD, as one might say) that was my optimistic viewpoint. Anything else we should just have to deal with as we could.

So, on the morning of the last day of that year, I re-read my "Molly's Memory" diary in its entirety. It made fascinating reading, but what really amazed me was how far back some of the events were, that I remembered as though they had happened this year. What did that say for my *own* memory?

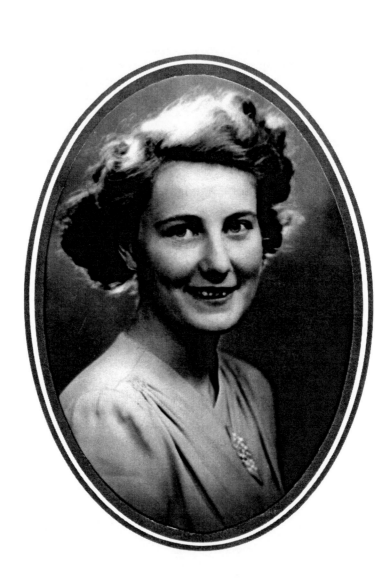

Engagement photo
1945

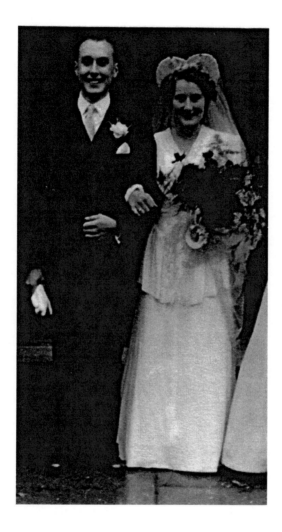

14 September 1946

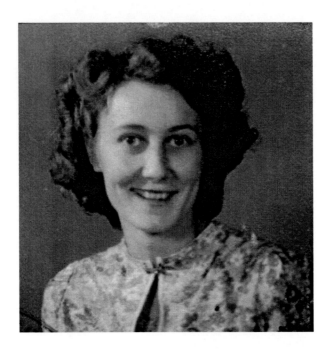

Passport photo 1948

One was allowed to smile
in those days

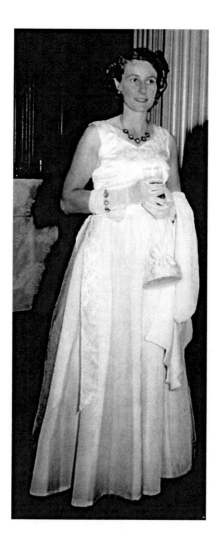

Molly at the opera.
Her ensemble was
sewn by her own
fair hand

CHAPTER 16

THE FUNNY FARM

The rest of the winter passed without much mishap, and my new life-arrangements meant that I did indeed have more time for Molly. Sometimes I brought her over to Carmelin for lunch and a dog walk, although the latter proved not always to be such a good idea. There was nowhere sheltered from the wind at The Lizard and Molly got cold, however warmly I dressed her, and complained long and loud.

"Isn't this horrible?" she said one afternoon as we battled our way along the lane, and she clasped her coat more firmly around her.

"Not too hot," I agreed. "Do you want to turn back?"

"No, it's all right." So we trudged on. But two minutes later she asked, "Isn't this horrible? Brrr! Where are we going now?"

"Just up the lane and around. Would you rather go home?"

"No, we'll carry on. Brrr!" So I walked faster, but all this did was keep me ahead of her a few steps, and another five minutes brought "This is horrible. Aren't we there yet?"

"No," I muttered into my scarf, pretending I couldn't hear her "but I wish we bloody well were!" This was not a process I enjoyed, and I concluded that it would be better for both of us if she were to forego my scintillating company and stay at home in the warmth.

A couple of days later I popped into Parc Bush and found Molly dressed to go out on her own, stuffing shoes and empty crisp packets into a bag and saying she was going to visit her mother. Unusually for me, I couldn't think of anything to say to stop her except the truth.

"Nan went to her reward ten years ago, Mother."

"What do you mean?"

"I mean she died."

"Did she? Oh well, it wasn't her I was going to see then." Molly stopped her bag packing and stood looking vague.

Having had a few seconds' thinking space, I changed the subject rapidly.

"Do you fancy a cup of coffee?" I dived into the cupboard and grabbed a packet of biscuits. "Have you tried these yet? They're really nice. I'll put the kettle on, shall I?" I gabbled. Once Molly was engaged in the fodder routine, sitting in the lounge with Tilly drooling at her feet, I made an excuse to go back to the kitchen and swiftly emptied her bag.

Poking around in my mother's handbag was not something that came naturally to me. Molly was such a private person, and in return would respect other people's privacy. I don't know of any other mother who, when dusting her teenage daughter's bedroom, would resist the temptation to read the diary at the bedside. But I had known, even at that young age, that she would not so much as open it, and I could happily leave it with its secrets undiscovered. Mother was the most upright, morally correct person I ever knew. She was no killjoy, and had a tremendous sense of humour and fun, but she adhered to the strictest of codes. Unfortunately, she expected everyone else to do the same, and felt severely let down when they didn't.

My father was undoubtedly one of Molly's greatest disappointments. He totally adored Molly, but, as they grew older together, they did not mellow and merge, but grew further apart. Although they moved to Cornwall in the early 1970's, Smithy continued to work in London from Tuesday to Friday, thoroughly enjoying his weekly train journeys and catching up with old friends in town in the evenings. His appearing in Cornwall only at weekends did not, however, help domestic matters. Although both he and Molly had thought it an ideal scenario, it soon became obvious that each was enjoying their freedom too much and finding it harder to accommodate the other's needs when they were together. About a year after moving down to Cornwall, they celebrated their silver wedding anniversary, and I asked Molly her views on matrimony after a quarter century of it. "Would you do it all again?" I asked.

"Get married, you mean?" she answered. "No, I don't think so. I'm too independent."

No-one could say she was not honest. My parents' marriage lasted another nine years in this barely tolerant fashion, Molly progressing through a very bad menopause, and Smithy having little time for sympathy. He was suffering his own problems at work, which eventually led to a nervous breakdown. Molly saw him through this - just - but could never understand that the work problems meant that Smithy had to go back to London to live. Doing what he had said he would never do, he asked her to return with him. Molly adhered to her black and white view of life. When they had discussed moving from London years before, she had said to him, "You'd better be sure you want this, because if I move to Cornwall, I am never coming back again!" She threw this at him now, and he had no answer, except to protest weakly that things had changed. She saw it as only *he* who had changed.

The inevitable happened and Smithy returned to London, bought a flat, and moved in permanently - alone. His last words to Molly, before he drove away, were, "I wish you would come with me."

So there you have it. Did he leave her, or did she leave him? How little it matters now ... but for one thing. Although all the experts will tell you that AD has nothing to do with stress, or emotional problems, it is also well known that the way we cope with stress has a bearing on how it affects us generally. Molly's only recourse to her problems was to get angry at Smithy, and we, her children, were not much help. If she used us as a sounding board for her anger, we could not reason with her, since defending him, or trying to bring in a different perspective, would only make her more cross, so we just made "Oh dear" responses, making her think that we were not even interested. Dysfunctional? You bet! A catalyst for AD? We are still guessing.

* * * * *

April came, bringing bright days, green buds, and seven baby pigs. Molly's paddock, neglected for over ten years, was going to be used by Sally and Martin to grow vegetables, but first it needed ploughing, and what better for the job than some little piggies? Afterwards, as a reward for their labours, they could be turned into sausages. So the piglets took up residence in the paddock, with *en suite* sty built by Martin, and a piglet-height electric fence to keep them in. This worked very well, and after the first shocking encounter they all kept well away from it. Tilly, however, curious as to what these little squeaky pink things were, trotted up to the fence one morning to have a look, connected with the wire and got the shock of her short life. Uttering a scream like a ... well, a stuck pig ... she took off from a standing start, raced past Martin who was bent double with laughter, down the field and through the garden. Sally, who was tidying the greenhouse, saw a doggy blur flash past her, came out to see what was happening, and was just in time to see Tilly crash through the hedge, and hear her yelps fade into the distance as she galloped off down the road. Tilly went so far and so fast that, by the time Sally had unlocked the gates, the dog was nowhere to be seen. Several hours' searching produced nothing, and Sally was just on the point of phoning the police when a kind neighbour rang and said he had found Tilly about half a mile from home. A few minutes later he brought her to Sally's door.

During all these hours, Molly did not once ask where Tilly was. Sally reported the whole story to me, and together we decided it was time to try an experiment. John and I would take Tilly to live with us for the next two weeks, and see if Molly missed her. Sad to say, she did not. I didn't deliberately keep her out of Molly's sight, so they met on several occasions, but if Molly asked "Where is the dog?" (she couldn't remember her name) I would just reply vaguely, "Oh, she's up the garden," or, if we were outside, "She's just gone indoors." Molly accepted this every time.

It was very sad that Molly, who would not so long ago have gone potty (sorry) at the thought of her dog going missing, now hardly noticed if she was there or not. If Tilly was nearby, then Molly would address the odd word to her - and of course would post cake into her mouth if given half a chance - but that was all. So Tilly started a cake-less life at Carmelin, and began to look better within weeks. Not so long before, when I was walking Tilly on Kennack Beach, a little girl spotted her, ran up to her father and cried, "Look, Daddy - a square dog!" But now that the pounds were falling off Tilly she was able to climb in and out of the car without heaving and puffing, and, most important of all for a dog, could turn her body into enough of a semi-circle to wash her parts.

Tilly missed Molly even less than Molly missed her, and totally accepted life with John and me. Her presence brightened each day for us, and even the cats seemed happy to have her around. A bonus for me was that, as Sally now didn't have to bother walking Tilly, I had Sundays off from visiting Molly. This might not sound like a politically correct reaction from a devoted daughter, but what bliss it was to wake up on a Sunday morning and know that I had the entire day to myself. And to be able to walk out of my own gate with Tilly for as long a walk as we fancied, without having to bundle her in and out of the car and worry about Molly fretting back at home over how long we'd been gone.

Back at Parc Bush - or, as we now termed it for obvious reasons, the Funny Farm - cake continued its star part in Molly's life. One of Martin's friends worked in a local bakery, where there was often stale cake left over at the day's end. Knowing that Martin kept pigs, he would donate the doughnuts to this worthy cause, and one afternoon he threw an entire bin-liner full of stale cakes, buns, pastries and scones over Molly's gate. Sally and Martin were out, so Molly got to it before they did, and must have thought it was her birthday. Sally found her on the kitchen floor, sorting her manna into piles, and when Sally protested that it was stale and some was mouldy, Molly replied frostily, "I *know*. That's why *that* pile is over *there*." So Sally left her to it and later on, when Molly was up the garden, Sally sneaked back indoors and retrieved the piggies' prandials.

Floors and fodder seemed to feature large in the lives of our ladies. Back in the US of A, Pob was on her knees in the kitchen one morning, rubbing a hunk of bread over the floor, when Jill walked in. Adrian reported:

> "What are you doing?" asked an incredulous Jill.
> "Cleaning the floor," replied Pob in an isn't-it-obvious? tone of voice.
> "Yes, but you're using bread!"
> Pob gave her a withering look. "I know," she said, and carried on scrubbing.

When I called on Molly soon after this and instigated the usual search for the handbag, I came upon a bag of stale buns that Sally had missed, lurking at the back of a kitchen cupboard. Some quick thinking was called for.

"Shall we go and feed the piggies, Molly?" I suggested. "Ooh look, here's some stale cake! We'll give them that and replace it with some new stuff later." As Molly walked out of the door with armfuls of rank bakery produce, I did a quick recce in the fridge in case the handbag had taken up residence there. It hadn't, but at the back, pushed between an empty saucepan and a tea towel, were three more dairy doughnuts, their cream tinged a delicate shade of blue-green. Even the pigs didn't need *that* much penicillin, so I stuffed the doughnuts into a plastic bag, threw it over the fence towards the dustbin, then hurried to join Molly on her path to the pigs. On my way out later, I collected the plastic bag and donated the doughnuts that night to the Carmelin fox. He'd been eating our leftovers, plus the occasional culinary failure, for years, so I knew he could cope with anything.

The bun run became a regular occurrence, and Sally got to know when to expect it and get out there before the cake queen. She got caught out once more though, and Molly hit the jackpot. Sally opened the fridge to look for milk, and found it crammed full of rock hard sponge cakes covered in gory red icing. An immediate invitation to the piggies' tea party was issued to Molly, and Sally garnered a handful of some of the less gooey numbers. Guiding Molly out of the door past a disappointed Martin who had been hoping for a cup of coffee, Sally thrust an empty box in Martin's hands and hissed, "Empty that fridge, quick!"

Sally now had a brilliant new routine in the mornings, going to Parc Bush first thing to feed the pigs and to check the newest additions to the Funny Farm, a flock of skinny, half feathered chickens, rescued from a battery farm. After seeing to these poor creatures who were learning to walk, to sunbathe and to peck in the dirt as Mother Nature had intended them to, Sally would have breakfast with Molly in the caravan and administer her pills. Incredibly, Molly would swallow these whole, sometimes without even a drink of water. Then Sally would say Cheerio-see-you-in-a-minute and Molly would happily amble off to watch the chickens, arrange flowers or meddle with anything she could find until someone else turned up.

On Tuesdays this was me, collecting my assistant for the shopping run. Molly enjoyed pushing the trolley while I piled stuff into it, and re-loading it with the packed bags I slid across to her at the checkout. As long as I kept her within my sight there were no problems, but I had learned my lesson the hard way one morning when there was a cold wind blowing. As we approached the doors, I told her to go and wait inside in the warm while I queued outside at the cashpoint. Having got my money, I went into the store but couldn't see her. With a cold feeling that had nothing to do with the weather, I experienced a moment of panic. I had lost my Mummy! Then I wondered "Did she actually go in?" and I looked outside. There she was, standing the other side of the entrance, obediently waiting for me, and oblivious to the chill wind blowing around her.

Once we had escaped, we would sit in the car, eating cheese pastries for elevenses and exchanging verbal inanities. After our shop, and having filled the car boot, I sent her off with the trolley to the trolley park as usual. Something made me look up seconds later, and there she was, nearly back at the main entrance. I had to run to catch her up.

"You don't have to go *that* far!" I puffed.

To which she replied, "Now you tell me!"

She had obviously got the taste for a long stroll. That evening, gale force winds made a mockery of our Fort Knox gates at Parc Bush, and blew so hard that the bolt was rattled right out of its socket and the gates opened wide. Molly made her escape. Fortunately she was found and rescued about a mile away, just before she reached the Helston road. I have to admit that my first thought was, "What a good thing *we* have Tilly now!" Well, maybe the second thought. Hell no, it *was* the first.

The next day, John and I had planned a day out, and so had Sally, so it was imperative that the gates held. John and I stopped on our way to check them. The bolt was holding but, to our dismay, we found Molly standing behind them, desperately trying to get out.

"Hullo! Where are you off to?" I enquired, as casually as I could.

"I'm going out," she snapped.

"I see." I had to dissuade her, but could think of nothing better than, "Well, why don't you wait until we come back? Then we can all go together."

"No!"

"*Why* do you have to go out?" A stupid question, but I was playing for time while I waited for my cerebrals to engage gear.

"There is someone up the road who might be nice to me."

It was no good arguing. Diversionary tactics were needed.

"OK, I'll come in. Let's go and check that everything's all right indoors, then we'll give you a lift."

My luck was in, and she accepted my suggestion. As we walked towards the house I started jabbering about food, pigs, garden - anything to distance her mind from escape - and it worked. She calmed down, and by the time we were indoors she had forgotten all about whoever it was who was going to be nice to her - not us, obviously! All this time, John was frantically tying up the gates with bits of string and some old washing line that just happened to be lying around, repairing the damage as best he could. When I thought he had had enough time, I made good my escape, telling Molly I had to go but would be back in half an hour. I exited swiftly before she decided to follow me, John letting me slip through the gates before tying the final knot, and we drove off.

The next day John returned and fixed a longer bolt on the outside of the gate. Yes, we were incarcerating my mother even more firmly in her own home. But, given the alternative of having her wander hither and yon, what choice did we have? The bolt held, the gate stayed shut from the outside, and Molly very soon lost interest in trying to get out at all.

There was still much to keep her amused inside. Besides the garden yielding endless material for her flower arranging, the house too was full of suitable ingredients. So, as well as having to check each vase and jar for posies well past their die-by date in rank, brown water, we also had to check for plates and dishes with an intermingling of anything that engaged Molly's magpie imagination: from flowers and leaves to slices of tomato, cheese and cake, often with a sprinkling of glass beads from necklaces she had picked apart. Her artwork was not so far removed from the creations that toddlers produce at playschool, or even those produced by professional artists for which gullible people will pay thousands of pounds, but it was the potential for putrification of Molly's work that bothered us. We developed a good diversionary tactic, sending her off to look for her handbag while we emptied as many vases as possible. One summer's day when Royce and Patti were making a rare visit, Molly had her back to the door while she spoke to them, and Sally walked in. Spotting a vase before she even closed the door, Sally picked it up, tossed the entire contents into the garden and put the vase back again. Patti couldn't believe her eyes. "What are you *doing*?" she mouthed. Then, realising, "I know; don't ask," and carried on chatting with Molly.

Molly was still quite capable of conversations at this time, and even if she couldn't find the right word, her brain - which was supposed to be atrophying - could come up with a new one. These were the early days of her language recall button not working so well, and my first recollection of it was when she showed me a plate with a crack in it.

"This is no good, it's got a great stronk right through it!" she said.

"Goodness me!" I replied. "I wonder how that happened?" There was a vague connection between the crack and "stronk", but this was just the start of Molly's New English Vocab. Often she would use the right word, in the wrong way, as when Sally found her in the caravan twiddling with something. "What are you doing?" she asked. "Taking the pies out," responded Molly, and when she looked closer Sally saw that she was cleaning her fingernails. On another occasion,

Sally was about to go and shut the chickens in for the night, when Molly asked, "Will I be able to brawn the lean?" Sally decided to be positive and answer in the affirmative. "Er, yes, I should think so," she replied, and went off, turning the question over in her mind as she tempted the chickens bedwards with a dish of corn. The answer was revealed when she came back in and found that Molly had indeed brawned the lean; she had pulled all the curtains in the caravan lounge.

Sometimes Molly would forget a word, usually a noun, but just substitute the word "thing". A common one was when we were out in the car, and she would point to the car in front, saying "Look at all the things he's got!" It took me several journeys to work this out. I would make the right noises, replying in automatic mode, "Gosh, yes! I wonder why he needs all those?" brain signals rushing uselessly from synapse to synapse trying to figure out what she meant, but the penny did not finally drop until we were waiting at traffic lights and she said, "Look at all those things! One, two, three ..." and by the time she had reached six I realised she meant the confabulation of traffic lights all showing red. Similarly, the "things" on the cars in front were their brake lights.

She also liked to read out the words painted on the road. "SLOW," would always make her giggle, which made me laugh too, but she would read "STOP" and not find it at all funny.

Basic reading was not a problem, but writing was another matter, and once again I had no idea until the evidence landed in my lap. On our way to the supermarket, I realised I had forgotten to put beer on the shopping list, so I asked Molly to do it. She managed to find the list and the pen in my bag and then asked me to repeat what it was I wanted her to write.

"Beer," I said.

"How do you spell that?"

I spelled it out slowly and she wrote it down in careful capitals as we drove along.   BBOR.

Oh ddor!

We enjoyed all sorts of other excursions too, always accompanied by a Molly commentary, and one spring bank holiday weekend John was doing a commentary of his own, loud-speakering for the car rally at a local Rotary fair, so I took Molly along. To anyone watching, it was a typical afternoon out with mother and daughter. She enjoyed the cars, the stalls and the displays, and, because she didn't say much, no-one would guess she had a problem. Her quietness worked well for her, hiding the confusion and blank spaces inside her head, so that she could appear quite normal.

Molly has always been quiet in company, even as a child. Her mother, Nan, was very chatty indeed, and tried to instil some of this social grace into her teenage daughter, telling her earnestly, "You must *speak* to people," to which the respectful daughter replied, "Well, of course, there's no need to when *you're* around, is there?" This silenced Nan for quite some time!

Emboldened by the success of the Rotary outing, Sally and I took Molly to the chiropodist in Helston. She had been once the year before, when Sally discovered several corns on Molly's feet (perhaps another reason for her thinking she was "not good any more" at walking) and had taken her, protesting, to have the corns removed. Now we were beginning to realise that, although Molly seemed quite clean and neat in her person, she was forgetting to take baths regularly, or to cut her toenails, and her nails looked so bad that we wondered if a blacksmith might be more appropriate. But we would try the chiropodist first, this time with both of us accompanying her. We needed the mutual moral support.

You would think we had dragged Molly to a torture chamber. It took several minutes' coaxing before we managed to get her into the chiropodist's chair, whereupon the perfectly charming young man fulfilled her worst fears, divesting her of shoes and silver lurex socks and proceeding to TOUCH her. Most people love having their footsies done, but not Molly. She doesn't like having her hair done either. Touchy she has no problem with, but touchy-feely never. Sally, Royce and I sometimes wonder how we arrived on this earth at all.

As Molly's socks made their exit, Sally and I looked at them and each other. "Bet she's had them on for three weeks," muttered Sally.

"Why don't you go down the road to a sock shop?" I murmured. So she did, while the lurid lurex walked into a plastic bag, and the chiropodist carried on valiantly through Molly's scowls, mumblings and foot twitchings.

Back came Sally ten minutes later with a big grin, flourishing three pairs of brand new socks. In pulsating pink or luminous lilac, each pair was embellished with a cartoon animal and embroidered slogan. The first had a cow and *Moooooooooody* as its motif; the second a pig and *Pigging Cheeky*; but the third pair was the one that, with much giggling, we decided upon, as it sported a sheep and *Baaamy*. Our giggles removed the stress from the operation, and we knew full well that Molly in her time would have done exactly the same with her own mother, and that Smithy would be looking down at us with a wry smile. Meanwhile our cheery chappy carried on smilingly, assuring us that he had seen much worse feet than Molly's. He should have been called a cheeropodist, so good naturedly did he perform his thankless task.

"But are other old dears as bad tempered as she is?" Sally enquired.

"Well, no" he smiled ruefully, "I've not had one *quite* this unhappy!" But he allowed us to make another appointment.

Over the next few months, Sally and I became increasingly aware of Molly's lessening interest in her person. She refused to buy new clothes, so I resorted to buying good quality charity shop offerings and giving them to her, pretending that they were my own cast-offs that didn't fit any more. Sally and I threw out an impressive number of Molly's rags, which had been clothes only in a former life, and encouraged her at every opportunity to change her outfit. Sometimes she would put on new ones of her own accord, but without taking off the first layer, and it took all our ingenuity to get her to change when she could see nothing wrong with her selection.

I also became what I never in my life thought I could be; Molly's personal hairdresser. Washing and cutting her hair myself actually proved easier than trying to take her to have it done professionally. The last time we had attempted this, I had nearly died of embarrassment at her rudeness to the hairdresser and her tuttings and twitchings as she tried to avoid the scissors. As for baths, she confessed to me that she "didn't bother with all that nonsense" any more; and the proof was in the tub. For months there had been not a drop of water, only dust. She did buy a bottle of bubble bath when we were shopping, which I found encouraging, but she had chosen it only because it was a pretty colour, and it sat on top of the cooker ever after.

It was not that she smelled or looked dirty (apart from her pre-chiro'd feet) but one would think that a lady who used to spend as long as possible in the tub every single day would carry on doing so. I mentioned it to our Amie, who suggested running the water and telling Molly, "Your bath is ready," but that too failed. Apart from this particular obstinacy, Molly enjoyed many sunnier moods and days, especially now that she had more company with the Ellises visiting every day. She would head for the caravan as soon as she saw Sally arrive, and particularly loved to watch the chickens, now well established in their run, from the window. She even noticed that there were more of them these days.

"My!" she exclaimed, jabbing her fingers in the air as she tried to count the chickens in their run, "look at all those clubits! One, two, three ..." She also loved to go out and talk to them, but by the end of the day she was often tired, and one evening, as some escapees milled around her feet, she became teasy and told them to go away. They didn't, of course, so Molly tutted in irritation and repeated her command. Spotting all this from the caravan, Sally leaned out of the window and said, "It's no good just saying 'Go Away'. You have to get close and tell them to bugger off!" So Molly leaned down and shouted at the poor things, "Bugger off!" and they did, legging it across the lawn with ruffled feathers and indignant squawks, while their audience laughed their socks off; which in Molly's case was probably a good idea.

I was by now doing all Molly's washing, clothes as well as sheets, managing a couple of machine loads a week, and thus feeling we were making some progress. Across the pond, however, Pob was still managing her own laundry. After a fashion.

> *Yesterday, when I got her home from "work", wrote Adrian, Pob decided that she was going to load up the machine. (This was an improvement on her attempt a couple of weeks ago when she tossed some dirty clothes in the trash bin, thinking that was going to wash them). She asked me how to make the machine start, so I told her that it was broken, and let her go on buggering around with it, knowing that while she was thus occupied, she wouldn't be sodding up anything else. But get this. I asked her if she had put any washing powder in, and she said that she never used it. Since the disinfectant episode, she probably hadn't, but a few minutes later I asked her again and she said that she had. So I asked her what she had used, since I knew that she had not opened the cabinet where the powder is kept. She opened the machine, yanked out a sheet of aluminium foil, and said, "There you are, I told you I put it in. This is washing powder, isn't it?" She never did get the machine started.*

One thing Molly did still manage to do was to feed herself, after a fashion. Since she had stopped using the cooker years ago (for which we were truly thankful) to fry her staple sausages and chips, she would instead just help herself to anything she fancied from the fridge. Now that we did our shopping together, and I chose all her food, she had a good selection, but Sally or I were not always present to administer it. Today, after frightening the chickens, Molly ambled off to forage, and appeared with a plate of neatly sliced cheese spread liberally with raspberry jam. One might laugh, but actually if you coated the cheese in breadcrumbs, shallow fried it, served it with a preserve, a frilly leaf and a drizzle of something, you could get away with charging £6.95 for it as a starter in a restaurant. Mmmm, delicious!

There was not much wrong with Molly's appetite. One morning, as Sally handed her a third piece of toast and marmalade, Molly exclaimed, "Oh goodness, I shall be bum bleck!" Sally wasn't quite sure that she had heard, so she said, "Pardon?" and, amazingly, Molly remembered long enough to repeat her words verbatim. We presume she meant either full up or fat as a pig. Or both.

But Molly's tastes were changing. This summer she drank her first cup of tea since 1945. I always thought she hated the stuff, but apparently she had told Sally that she drank so much of it during the war that, when peace came, she vowed she would drink no more, and she didn't. Until this summer. What was even stranger was that she asked for sugar with it. We had never known her to take sugar in her coffee, and the reason she gave for this was that she couldn't get *any* during the war. So make of that what you will.

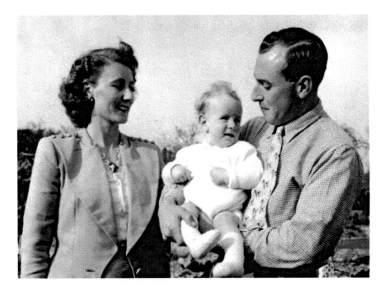

Molly, Royce, Alan. April 1954

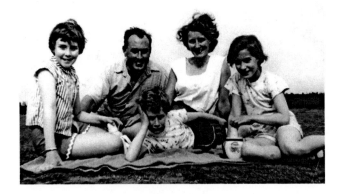

Sally, Alan, Royce, Molly, Jane
1959

Sally, Jane, Ruby, Royce, Molly.
1954

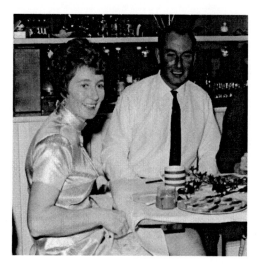

Molly and Smithy. Christmas 1969

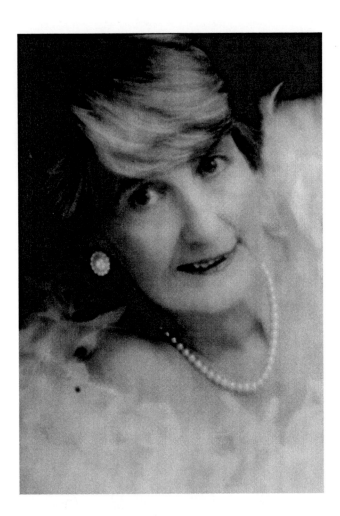

Molly's "Hollywood Portrait"
1988

113

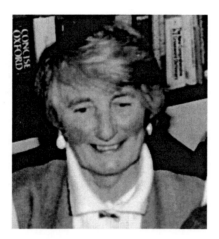

November 1993

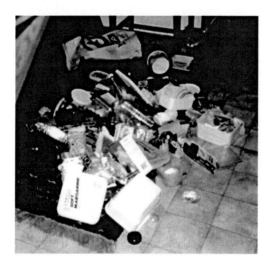

Contents of Molly's fridge
and cupboards (not
including the cat).
June 2002

CHAPTER 17

THE EVEN FUNNIER FARM

By July 2004, Sally and Martin were starting to move home. This was a relaxed process at first, with Sally carefully packing up one box each day, wrapping china, books, ornaments and kitchen equipment in layers of newspaper and bubble wrap, then transporting it at her leisure to Parc Bush. On site, the caravans were installed, connected to the mains water and ready for occupation. Under the supervision of our supposedly retired builder friend Dudley (Norma's husband, and AD-Mavis's son in law), the paddock witnessed the installation of a huge bulbous sewage tank, known as an onion. I could imagine Molly, in her sparkier days, saying that a sewage tank was the best place for onions, but it was a system reputed to be cheaper and easier than connecting the caravans to the mains sewerage. I had my doubts, and future bills proved enough to scare the sewage out of anyone, but there it was.

Martin had also done a magnificent job of connecting the two caravans with a covered walkway, so that he and Sally and the girls could go back and forth on rainy days without getting wet and muddy. This project happened to coincide with the local builders' merchants being taken over by a larger conglomerate, and there was a lot of reorganising going on in their yard, with much surplus material being dumped. Martin was in the yard one day, looking for something, and saw a skip heaped high with odd pieces of wood, plasterboard and hardboard.

"Throwing that out, are 'ee?" he asked of an employee.

"Yes, mate, got no use for that. Gotta tidy up the place for the new bosses!"

"Well, how much do you want for it?"

"For that lot? You can 'ave 'ee for nothin'. Glad to get rid of it."

Martin needed no further encouragement, and, after that, every time he turned up with his truck, a load of very useful rubbish was transferred to it from the skip, sometimes for free, sometimes for a few pounds, and once he was back home, like the proverbial blind man, he picked up his hammer and saw. The result was a little à la shanty-town, but it did the job. What was more, once his friends saw the creation, word spread round the village that the Ellises were grateful for donations, and all sorts of stuff would turn up in the front yard of Parc Bush. Old carpets, chairs, sofas, kitchen cupboards, double glazed windows; it was much easier for folk to donate to the Ellis cause than to drive their rubbish to Helston dump twelve miles away. A simple caravan walkway developed into a kitchen extension, back porch, freezer room, cloakroom, workshop and Martin's personal lounge complete with home-brew bar.

The only thing missing was a fire, but that was soon fixed. Since Molly had finally stopped using her wood-burner, Martin moved it out of her lounge and into his own, and we bought Molly a very convincing electric version. Moving a wood-burner is not the sort of thing a fisherman does every day, but it all seemed to slot into its new home quite well, including the chimney, its base buried under several inches of fire cement. That evening, once Molly was safely ensconced in bed, several of Sally and Martin's friends came along to witness the ceremonial lighting of the fire and settled down for a cosy night's beer drinking and ciggie smoking. Before long, however, in an excess of companionable camaraderie, the fire started smoking too, emitting smouldering puffs every few seconds from the joint where chimney joined stove. Martin closed the doors more firmly but to no avail; he opened the damper but the chimney belched forth even more thickly. It was one of Martin's friends, who had a wood-burner of his own, who suddenly said, "There's your trouble, mate. You've got the chimney on upside down!"

"Flippin' 'ell!" exclaimed Martin, and everyone sprang into action. Sally rushed outside and fetched the wheelbarrow, the guys grabbed the fire-irons and pulled burning logs from the fire, throwing them into the barrow which Sally pushed at a run back down the corridor and out into the garden, her long blonde hair streaming out behind her as she raced across the grass, her mobile bonfire throwing out clouds of ash and sparks at every bump.

By the time he had re-fixed it a day or so later, Martin was a well qualified installer of wood-burners.

In future months, friends would flock to Martin's lounge, often after the pub closed, bringing a bottle with them, and the party would continue until all hours. Because of the novelty of having a b-y-o bar on a pig farm, it was named The Tiddly Pig, and was a great success for several seasons, right up until the time the law changed, permitting the village pub also to remain open all hours.

Now, the only thing holding Sally and Martin back from moving in full time to the caravans was the lack of electricity. Since our good friend Charlie had departed for the joys of Essex, Dudley was trying to arrange for another electrician to take over. This chap was still busy doing sharp intakes of breath at another job, so we had to wait. And wait. But Sally and Martin could at least spend most of their daytime hours at Parc Bush and had already moved their pets into Molly's garden and field. So now, as well as seven pigs and twenty chickens, there were also three rabbits and two guinea pigs. Molly, an animal lover all her life, was in her element. The star guinea pig was Rasdus, a handsome fellow with ginger biscuit fur so long and lustrous that he was dubbed a guinea wig. Then, next to the guinea pigs' cage, came their neighbours from hell, mum and dad ferret plus seven sweet but smelly kits.

One day Martin picked up a road-killed rabbit on his travels and brought it home to feed to these voracious little carnivores. He threw it into their pen and they fell upon it. This greatly distressed Molly who was standing watching, obviously thinking the rabbit was still alive.

"Leave it alone!" she instructed them through the wire of their run. "Stop it!"

"They won't take any notice of you, Molly," pronounced Martin. "That's their dinner!"

"Yes, but they're ... oh ... *leave it!*" And she rattled the wire. The ferrets looked up, momentarily startled, one of them with a piece of fur dangling from its chops, then dived once more into the bunny body.

"Don't worry, Molly," soothed Martin. "The rabbit's dead."

"Is it?" said Molly, not quite convinced. She took one last glance before leaving the scene and forgetting all about it. Or so we thought. Later that evening Sally and Martin found the ferrets running loose in the guinea pig run, bellies bulging, and with nothing left of dear Rasdus but a few strands of long, ginger hair. Sally was beside herself. What could have happened? Her investigation soon told her. A pair of secateurs in Molly's kitchen, a large hole cut in the side of the ferrets' run, and no sign of the rabbit carcass. Obviously the ferrets had had their rabbit supper removed, lost no time in finding an alternative, and Molly was the culprit. I am sorry, but this was one occasion when I found it hard to accept the peculiarities of AD and was quietly furious.

We regained our sense of humour later in the day, when Martin and a pal were moving a fridge into the shed, as one does, and pal leaned down to pick up an upside down bucket that was in the way. He dropped the bucket with a shriek while everyone else fell about laughing as they saw, hidden underneath it, the half eaten corpse of the aforementioned rabbit. Well, at least the bunny had had a speedy demise. And the ferrets got seconds.

Towards the end of August, the electrics still not completed, Sally and Martin moved into the caravans at last, having had the golden opportunity of letting their house to a family who were desperate for accommodation. They would be. Their party consisted of one man, his woman, four children by her previous husband, a baby from one of these offspring, and the woman's own baby from the present partner. They said they would take the house, whatever condition it was in, never mind the cleaning and a bit of scratched paint, as long as it was NOW. They concluded their request by offering a fistful of cash. Who could resist?

Within twenty four hours Sally had called in the troops and we were marching. Molly was always happiest when actively involved, so I collected her on my way to Sally's house and she helped too, cleaning anything that was going to be left behind. She got on very well, except that there was a substantial amount of dust in the air, and it was making her sneeze. "Ooh," she sniffed, "I must get a cattiper." "Here you are," I said, passing her a tissue. "Have one of mine." All family cars were commandeered as removal lorries, and the contents of the house that had not already been shifted in Sally's orderly fashion were thrown into any container available, squashed into the nearest vehicle and driven the half mile to Parc Bush.

We all worked steadily, with only the occasional break to feed cake to Molly and ourselves, but by early evening had run out of boxes, bags, time and energy. Desperate, I put through a frantic "Help!" phone call to John in his office at home, and ten minutes later he turned up on Sally's front door step, looking quite the part in his green baize pinny and clutching a sackful of carrier bags. He crammed his car with all the Ellis belongings I threw at him, whilst I completed my own final load including Bella the cat, yowling in protest at being basketed, and Clem the dog, always ready for a ride. Thus the final convoy wound its way to Parc Bush. I wished I'd had the camera to take a picture of John later, leaning on his laden car amongst the chaos in Molly's garden, still in his pinny, mobile phone to his ear and talking high finance to a business colleague.

I don't think I will ever forget the sight of a string of cars along Molly's garden, and a trail of worldly goods strewn just everywhere. The place looked like Ma and Pa Larkin's farm, only without the darling buds. We had started by trying to find sensible places to put stuff, but soon gave up. Cars drove to and fro across the lawn while boxes, suitcases, bin liners and overflowing carrier bags were piled high in caravans, house, shed and garden, surrounded and topped off by yet more things that had not been lucky enough to be packed, and all in severe danger of toppling onto each other at any moment. Thank goodness it was a dry night, so the only thing we had to worry about was Molly meddling, which she did with great thoroughness. Sally and Martin's belongings turned up over the following months in all sorts of odd places, and some, just like Charlie's cable, never surfaced at all.

Over the next few weeks Molly revelled in her new-found companionship, and the activity around her worked some minor miracles. She was happier, calmer, and even improved in her speech, remembering words she had forgotten and stringing sentences together better. It seemed, however, that the balance of companionship and independence was a delicate one, and this raised an interesting comparison with Pob around this time, of whom Adrian wrote as follows:

Today Jill is attending a seminar, which means that she has to be out by seven thirty in the morning, too early for her usual routine of getting Pob ready for "work".   When Jill is around, Pob becomes much more helpless (just like the rest of us when we can rely on someone else), but when Jill is not available, the old girl rallies considerably and helps herself. Pob has always been a sharp dresser, and this morning she got herself washed, completely dressed, make-up on and fastening a necklace. As far as I could see, she got everything right. The only help she needed was getting her bra strap hooked up. (Ugh. She is about a half century too late for those tricks, and in any case my forte was always un-hooking 'em ... but I digress). There was a helluva lot more of the old personality and sense of humour there this morning.

Molly was still able to dress herself at this stage, getting it right most of the time, but we knew that her temporary improvement was, sadly, only a blip, and it was not long before another AD first occurred. During the first weekend in their new home, Martin and Sally were having a relaxing morning cuppa in bed in the caravan, when Martin happened to look out of the window at the view across the garden. "Uh-oh," he said. "This is going to shorten our time here."

"What do you mean?" asked Sally.

"Well, as soon as Molly has to go into a home, we have to find somewhere else to live."

"That's right. And ... ?"

"Molly's bringing the washing in. And she seems to have forgotten to put her trousers on."

Sally took a peek. Molly was happily picking the washing off the line, and was dressed in a nice warm coat and a pair of tights and shoes, but sure enough, no trousers. Sally shook her head, but carried on drinking her tea. She had a feeling that Molly's trouserlessness was to be the least of their troubles.

For the time being, Molly's foibles were minor. She continued conversing with the chickens and feeding them scraps – sometimes bread and cake, sometimes lumps of polystyrene - and the wild birds got a similar variety – one day cheese, the next soap powder. She kidnapped Bella, shutting the cat in the upstairs bathroom, and getting quite heated when Sally tried to take the poor thing back again. We were not sure what to do about this, but Bella gave her own answer, moving into the house of her own accord and taking up permanent residence on Molly's bed. Clem too loved to go indoors, and would lie on the cool kitchen lino, panting and being fed with cake. Or he would follow Molly devotedly round the garden while she was bringing in Sally's washing – dry or not - and putting it where Sally couldn't find it; a stack of neatly folded towels in the study, for instance, and frilly knickers of all different colours in the fridge. One day I gave her a clean pair of socks to wear and she put them on her hands.

None of Molly's idiosyncrasies were life-threatening. We just had to be a little more patient than normal, and in that respect they taught us a valuable lesson. We had learned not to be surprised at what she did, and we involved her in the laughter if we could. There was so much of it. Sometimes Molly could be irritating, but she seldom meant to be, and sometimes she was just plain hilarious. Much of the work on and around the caravans, even after they were installed and occupied, involved a mini JCB making a mess, and Molly understandably hated this. Of course we could not reason with her, so, given enough notice, I would bring her back to Carmelin with me for a few hours while the work progressed. However, the driver turned up at Parc Bush unexpectedly one afternoon and engaged himself in making even more chaos than usual with his digger, gouging gatepost holes and levelling out ground, serenely unaware of Molly watching him through narrowed eyes.

"You bugger!" she muttered vituperatively. "You silly old fool!"

Sally overheard this and took great delight in telling the driver later that Molly had called him a bugger.

"Arr well," he grinned, "she'm roight there!"

Life gradually settled into a semblance of routine, and on 26 August Molly celebrated her 79th birthday. We bought her a battery operated toy cat that mioawed and purred, turned its head, twitched its tail and all but ate lunch. Molly loved it. She would make it comfortable on a chair, cover it with a blanket, and engage it in earnest cat-conversation. Sally, treating herself to a bath in the bungalow one morning, was serenaded by a cats' chorus of miaows from both the cat and Molly. This batteried feline was tucked up in a nest of cushions at night, whilst Bella, the real thing, plus any amount of stuffed toys, snuggled up to her new mum in bed. As summer drew to its golden close, Molly was a happy bunny.

* * * * *

In a moment of reflection, I could not help thinking that, nearly six decades earlier, she had been even happier. September 14th marked 58 years since Molly and Smithy's wedding. How many of us, on such a joyful occasion, would be able to see what the future held? Or even want to? Those two young people, each only 21 years old, beautiful and blessed, held the world in the palm of their hands, and could see only the years of happiness ahead, and none of the sad endings that were to follow. I thanked providence for the resilience and sense of humour with which they conquered any troubles, and which they passed on to us, their children.

Perfection it was not, but my parents' marriage was basically a happy one. Their separation, when Smithy went back to London, lasted only a few years, by which time he was wishing with all his heart that he could turn back the clock. Wishes in this case proved to be horses, and when he and Molly were thrown together semi-socially (it was at the funeral of a mutual friend in London), Smithy nervously suggested to Molly that they get back together again. To the delight of us all, including friends, distant family - heck, *the world* - she agreed, and came back from the funeral on cloud nine. She and Smithy had four more years together after this, including their ruby wedding anniversary, before Smithy was claimed to go to his reward.

Molly's reaction to her sudden widowhood was, I have to say, interesting. As I had, of course, lost my dad, I asked her which was worse - losing her husband or losing her father.

"My father," she replied without hesitation. This would undoubtedly have something to do with the fact that her father's death, from a stroke, had been a complete shock, whereas she had had weeks, if not months, to get used to Smithy being mortally ill. She was also, as I have mentioned before, introverted in character, and Royce asked me a few days after the funeral, "Do you think Mother actually loved Dad?"

"Oh yes," I replied without hesitation. "She just didn't show it to others." Besides being sure of this because I knew Molly well, I had it from Smithy himself. "She might not show it," Smithy said of Molly, "but she certainly feels it."

A few years later, when Nan died, Molly's feelings were further revealed when someone commented to her how upset she must be.

"I suppose it is sad," replied Molly unconvincingly, "but nothing has been able to touch me since Alan died."

All the experts will tell you that AD has nothing to do with emotions or stress, but I wonder, I really do.

* * * * *

Molly's new improved mode continued on its erratic course in the summer of 2004. Sally and I took her on a girly shopping trip to town, intending to buy her a new jacket, and the three of us had as much fun as we used to in the old days. Although at first she said she didn't want to try on any coats, we employed the usual tactic of leaving it for a few seconds, then approaching the task from a slightly different angle and trying again. Eventually, we got her to try on several, so I got some idea of what suited her, and when she still insisted that she didn't want a new one, I pretended to buy one for myself, which I would give to her later. I did well from this deal, as she proclaimed she liked my old red one better, so she had that instead, and I kept the new one.

All shopped out, we proceeded to the Tea Rooms for sustenance. The home-made cake was delicious, but my coffee was very bitter, and eventually, in spite of my ladling copious amounts of sugar into the cup, I could drink no more. Not wanting to upset the proprietress, I turned to Sally.

"Can I pour this into your teapot?" I whispered. "I don't want her to think I don't like it."

"No!" replied Sally indignantly. "She'll think that *I* don't like my tea!"

I tried Molly. "Would you like some more coffee, Mother?"

"No, thank you."

I sighed, waited a few seconds, then poured half of my cup's contents into hers. She drank it, so I poured in the rest, with extra milk, and she took another sip.

"Ugh!" she said, and pushed it away. Ten minutes later, as we got up to go, I pushed the cup back at her, and asked, "Don't you want this?"

"Oh," she said, "I didn't realise I'd left it," and drank the lot.

So, OK, I am a cruel and conniving daughter, and John says I took advantage of the poor old lady. I suppose I did, but in my defence she has never eaten or drunk anything she doesn't like, Alzheimer's or no Alzheimer's.

She continued to surprise us with her changing tastes, though. Not only had she started to drink tea again, but one October day Sally phoned me with some special news.

"You'll never guess what Molly's doing!" she said.

"Oh God. What now?"

"She's eating stew."

"But she doesn't like stew! Has it got vegetables in?"

"Yes; onions, garlic and carrots." None of which Molly had touched in her life.

"Blimey," was all I could think to say.

"And she's listening to a pop group on the tape player."

"Which pop group?"

"'Madness'," giggled Sally.

"Oh, you are awful!" And another AD moment was lightened.

It was as well that Sally was starting to include Molly in the family mealtimes. During November Molly had a couple of dizzy spells, saying, "I feel all funny," and waving her hands about. We rushed her off to the doctor to have her blood pressure checked, but it was fine, and Sally concluded that lack of food might have been the problem. Although Molly would eat like a horse during the day, she went to bed so early, often as soon as it got dark, that sometimes she simply forgot to feed herself in the evening. So Sally started to make suppertime sandwiches for her, plus an orange and a piece of cake, delivered while Molly lay in bed fully clothed, surrounded by her stuffed toys and with Bella-cat cuddled up to her, purring happily. Molly would tuck in gratefully, offering the occasional nibble to the cat. Bella politely declined but, judging from the funny colours we noticed around their mouths, Molly was more insistent with the toys.

Sandwich-making seemed to be a family talent. Opening a drawer in the kitchen one morning to put in some clean tea-towels, I encountered four pieces of bread and butter laid neatly in the drawer, each with six tiny cheese biscuits, also buttered, placed precisely on top. "Is someone coming round to tea?" I asked Molly and she grinned, seeing the funny side because she does, and also because she no doubt thought that somebody else had done the deed.

She thought the same when I noticed an upturned flowerpot of mud in Sally's egg collecting basket by the back door. "Have you been making mud pies?" I asked Molly, but she could remember nothing about it, and just shook her head in puzzlement at the strange sight.

Molly's moods were so sunny these days that I managed to get her into the bath three times in as many weeks. This had, nevertheless, taken a deal of prior thought and cunning. Since Amie's suggestion of running the bath and then calling Molly to it had been an immediate failure, I thought briefly of Norma's approach with Mavis, who, in spite of her night-time attempts to boil herself alive, had done all in her power to avoid water at other times. Norma had succeeded with quiet insistence - all right, bullying - but I knew this would not work with Molly. So I coaxed her into the tub with promises of going out to tea afterwards. This succeeded brilliantly for a while. If I had time, we did go out afterwards; if not, she forgot my promise before she even stepped onto the bath mat, and although this left me with guilt feelings, it was not for long. It was more important that we keep Molly clean.

During that first bath-time, I left Molly to do everything herself while I respectfully hung around outside, listening for the splashing noises, and handing her clean clothes through an arm's width of open door. This modest approach seems odd now, but after 54 years of not seeing my mother in anything less than a swimsuit, it was quite a barrier to overcome to actually undress her. But only for me. She was completely unperturbed to be assisted in divesting herself of her clothes, and soon I was doing it without thinking.

In Virginia, Pob was experiencing her own bathroom triumph.

A couple of days ago, wrote Adrian, *she tried to flush her toilet in the morning, and nothing happened because the bit of chain that goes from the flush handle to the flapper in the tank had come off. So she told me and I promised to fix it. Well, I forgot, and the toilet was still out of action in the evening when I brought Pob home from her "job". When she disappeared into the bathroom, I knew that she would have forgotten that she had told us about it in the morning, so I decided to make the most of that and would pretend to be surprised when she said that she couldn't flush the bog. She was in there a helluva time, but I heard some clanking and clattering going on, so I knew she was still alive, and then she came out and announced, with a tone of triumph in her voice, "Well, that's done! I got tired of waiting for you, so I damn well fixed it myself." I didn't even know that she knew what the inside of a toilet tank looked like!*

There are no rules with AD. Just when you think you have got "it" worked out, Molly or Pob will astound you with something clever or witty, as their old selves momentarily flash into view once more. Sometimes this can be even more disturbing than the steady downward trend, but one thing Sally and I were cottoning onto was the fact that music would goad the memory cells into action swiftly and accurately. Molly would hum along to any musicals she recognised on television or video, and this did make things easier for us at times. As another year drew to a close, and Christmas came round again, I volunteered to be in charge of Molly's entertainment schedule. There wasn't going to be much, since, having been ill for several days before Christmas, I did not have a great store of mental strength or patience. However, I fetched Molly late in the morning and settled us down by a roaring fire in the sitting room, switched on the classically brilliant video of Showboat, gave Molly a plate piled high with turkey sandwiches and mince pies, and put a stack of presents by her side for her to unwrap - soap, hankies, toys, sweets, a simple jigsaw puzzle - all the sorts of things she would delight in and which should keep her amused for ages.

Soon Molly was humming happily as she nibbled at her victuals, so I crept out of the lounge, fetched John and Tilly, and locked the back door while we went for a short walk. Unkind? I don't think so; she was far happier doing what she was doing. Our little ruse did nearly backfire, though. Because I was only ambling, the walk took John and me more time than we had planned, whilst the video took less, and by the time we returned it had finished and we found Molly wandering in the kitchen. We were just so relieved that we had taken the double precaution of locking all doors. I switched the box back on for our traditional viewing of The Snowman, and I then took Molly home before dark.

All in all it was a good day for Molly, but I was glad for once that her memory was so bad. Had she been able to remember the Christmases of our childhood, and indeed her own, she could not have helped but make a sad contrast. Now, once she was back in her home, in her bed, with cat and toys, Molly forgot what she had been doing forty seconds ago, never mind forty years, and went to sleep.

CHAPTER 18

SHOPS AND SHAMPOOS

2005 did not start well. Sally's house tenants finally found a larger house to wreck, and moved out, leaving the house looking like a tip. In the kids' bedrooms every wall was covered in graffiti, most of it not the sort of words that dear little children should know; or indeed elderly mothers, so, when Sally and Martin's army of cleaners moved in once more, we left Molly at home. The job was fun for a while, but my fluey bug was still clinging on tenaciously, and I found the whole task exhausting. But we kept doggedly on, slapping on emulsion in any shade we could find (Molly's shed was a real treasure trove) from brilliant turquoise to apricot custard. It didn't put off the prospective tenants, and a new couple soon moved in.

Sally and Martin's kindness in looking after Molly was now being rewarded; at least they had somewhere to live. But the Ellis troubles were not yet over. Martin's fishing was still not going well, his boat becoming the proverbial hole in the water into which he poured money, and now, to add injury to insult, his knees were giving way. Having spent their lifetime balancing his burly body on a bobbing boat, they had finally creaked to a standstill. The Fishermen's Mission hospital in London put him on their waiting list for two separate knee replacement operations, but there was no telling when this might happen. The storm which had been clouding the horizon for months was now upon him. He had to give up fishing and sell his boat.

However, the ill wind was blowing some good. As he put it succinctly, "I no longer have to get up at 4 a.m. to go out in the frigging cold and wind to try and catch fish that aren't there, wasting my time, energy and money on a hopeless cause. I can stay at home and concentrate on my gardening."

And he did. The piggies were dispatched (don't ask; you don't want to know), the tractor chugged into view once more, the paddock was ploughed, potatoes were sown, and Martin's leisure time reading changed from Fishing News to seed catalogues. He spent his days slowly but surely cultivating the paddock, and, as spring approached, Parc Bush Gardens were showing signs of becoming the organic vegetable centre for Ruan Minor.

Other produce, of course, had to come from town, so Molly and I continued to do the weekly run. The routine was easy and fun, but another sad surprise awaited me when Molly asked, for the first time ever, which side of the car she should get in.

"The passenger side," I replied, adding jokily, "unless you want to drive?" This ignored the scary fact that she actually still had (has!) a current driving licence.

Having sat her in the passenger seat, my routine was always to hand her the seat belt, and say, "Put that in the red thing," and without fail she would push it into my clip, instead of hers. But now she surprised me again, still putting it into my clip, but actually noticing and saying before *I* did, "The wrong one!". Then she looked around Wenna's car parked in front of us and warned me as I pulled out, saying, "Look out, here comes a car." She was also lucid enough to look left when we stopped at a junction and say, "OK my way." Yes, I did check, but she hadn't got it wrong. Driving along, we encountered a very slow car in front. "Hurry up!" we both said at the same time - and he did. "Oh, he must have heard us," said Molly. Her composure deserted her at the traffic lights, however, when the car in front was slow in pulling away. "Come on, you squitter!" she barked.

I hardly need add that this term is now firmly rooted in our family patois.

I found it interesting that the hurry-up trait was shared by Pob. Adrian told me:

> *Every day when I take her to "work", or bring her home, she is always talking to the bloke in the car in front, telling him to hurry up and move along a bit faster. Damn good job she isn't driving. As a matter of fact, a couple of days ago she said that it was about time she started driving again. I'm not worried - I have heard stuff like that so many times now that I know the thought will be gone in three or four minutes.*

Back on the road to Helston there would be innumerable chatterings from Molly where I didn't have a clue what she was talking about, but once inside the supermarket she was more focused, and we spent much of our time along the aisles, especially the vegetable section, giggling while she said Urgh, and I said You-wouldn't-like-this.

Sometimes the old Molly, with her sparky sense of fun, would come up with a real gem. Spying a notice on the cheese counter, she read fluently, "Bargains on your doorstep," and added, "shall we go home, then?" Then something caught her attention at the spaghetti shelves and she pulled at my sleeve, saying,

"Have you seen this?"

"What?" I asked, expecting to see a large, colourful notice, but there was nothing.

She continued, "You can see it and read it, and then bury it for a short while."

I paused not one second before replying, "Oh yes! So you can! I never noticed."

I still have no idea what she meant.

Sometimes the giggling would stop. I met a friend of John's and mine in the wine aisle and we stopped for a chat while Molly stood quietly by. A few minutes later, as we queued at the checkout, he passed us again. Fortunately he had just passed out of earshot when Molly threw him a filthy look and said, "Silly fool!" I don't know what he was supposed to have done, so I said, "That's my friend you are talking about!" Molly just shrugged.

We ate our elevenses as usual in the car park, and headed home. Molly finished her bun as we drove, folded the plastic wrapper neatly and pushed it down her glove. Then she took it out again and used it as a handkerchief. "Oh, that's no good," she said, looking at it with some distaste.

"I should think not!" I replied. "Here, have this," and I fished a tissue out of my pocket not quite in time to stop her wiping her nose on her glove. Then on the tissue.

"Do you want it back?" she asked.

"No thank you!"

"No, I thought not." A few seconds later I looked down to see her rolling her trouser above her knee and pushing the tissue down her pop-sock. What I was not expecting to see was a foot of pink chiffon scarf protruding from her trouser leg. We both laughed at the same time, and I exclaimed "I wondered what on earth you were doing!"

"So did I!" she replied, rolling her trouser leg back down - but not in time to hide the fact that two pieces of pink toilet tissue were tucked into the pink scarf. At least she was colour co-ordinated.

It seems to me that the AD mind goes particularly AWOL when left alone, but can sometimes be called to attention later. Hence the (unreasonable) donning of scarf and tissue paper, followed by the (reasonable) surprise at finding it. This reminded me of when my father was in hospital during the last months of his life. High on morphine, he would "see" all sorts of oddities, perhaps a black cat climbing over the window sill, or a nurse with a Kango hammer; and he would mumble and mutter in a half-dream world. Then, if one engaged his attention, he could talk for ages on any subject quite comprehensibly. Molly could not talk for very long these days, but she could understand what I said to her, and accompany me round a shop quite sensibly. However, the vocabulary and identification skills were definitely fading. So often, when we were looking for something she would find something else. Look for a glove and she would offer a towel; say you needed a hanky and she would give you a flower. Her speech was noticeably declining and we often had a reverse of the toddler syndrome where only the mother can understand her child. Sally and I became the "parents" but, unlike a child, Molly's needs would increase and her capabilities and vocabulary would lessen.

Bath time was another toddler problem. I had been really pleased with myself only a few months before when I had often been able to tempt her into the bath with the prospect of going out for coffee and cake afterwards, but my success had been short-lived. She now complained so loud and long about the cold when I tried to get her in the bath, in spite of it being springtime and the fan heater going full blast, that I gave up for a couple of weeks. Then, when I did succeed, I was alarmed to see pale purple blotches on her knees, her front and the small of her back. Her fingers were a similar colour but, when I felt them, did not seem unusually cold, so I decided not to panic just yet.

Sally and I checked on Molly's colour the next day, and her blue blood seemed less blue than before, and the blotches faded away over the next few days, so we concluded that it must have been a mix of less than perfect circulation and a cool spell of weather. When Sally asked her, "How are you today?" Molly replied, "I'm manging" (to rhyme with banging), and her accompanying facial expressions seemed to indicate that this was a positive experience.

There seemed to be nothing physically wrong with her, and this was borne out one fine day when she escaped from Parc Colditz and went walkabout for the first time in a year. We could only conclude that someone must have left the gate open, for it would only take a matter of minutes for Molly to spot it and wander off. Sally despatched the girls as a search party, in Wenna's car, but some neighbour found Molly within minutes and delivered her back home.

"Wait till your father gets home!" scolded Sally, as she opened the gates, but for once Molly did not appreciate the humour. She gave one of her shrugs and flounced off indoors.

Because of this escapade, Sally was nervous for a while about leaving Molly alone. So, one day, when both Sally and Martin needed to be out, I brought Molly to Carmelin. John was just coming out of his office as we arrived, but when he saw us, that look of panic came into his eyes and he only managed a brief "Hi!" before remembering an urgent something he had forgotten, and diving back in.

"It's not catching, you know!" I flung after him, as I helped Molly up the step into the kitchen, shaking my head and smiling in spite of myself. The poor guy just did not know what to *say*. I settled Molly in the sherb where I could keep an eye on her through the French doors from my office, and gave her a colourful magazine. Within minutes she came in and interrupted me.

"Can I do ...?" and she mumbled something unintelligible. I didn't know what it meant, but whatever it was, I was busy. So I permitted myself, just for once, to be firm with her and replied, "No, I have to do this first."

"Oh," she said, "well, can you be quick, because I want to get rid of this," and her hand strayed in the area of her posterior. Oops! Did I feel bad! I almost fell off my chair in my haste to get her to the bathroom. Then she needed to go twice more during the morning. Goodness knows what Café Ellis had been feeding her.

In the afternoon I had planned to walk Tilly, but I wasn't sure how far Molly could walk and whether I should take her with me or leave her at home. I suggested various alternatives to John, but his face resumed that look of alarm and he could only say, "I'll do anything you want, but don't leave Molly with me!" So Tilly and I took her along with us and we had quite a nice amble around the coastal paths. We then sat in the lounge, but she couldn't seem to settle to anything, whatever I gave her to do. Scrapbooks, photo albums, jig-saw puzzles - nothing held her attention. She just wanted to take the pictures out of the albums, or wander around and fiddle with things. Fortunately Martin collected her quite soon, and I am ashamed to say that my only emotion was relief. I just could not do what he and Sally were doing. I would be hysterical within days.

We were missing out on the fun though. Back at Parc Bush, Molly found a photo album which contained pictures of her childhood friends and she took it into Wenna and Toana's caravan. "I thought you might like to see this," she said.

"Thank you," they said and politely turned the pages with her. When they had finished, she took the album, stood up to go, then turned back to them.

"Have you seen this?" she asked, and thrust the book at them upside down. The girls collapsed into immediate hysterics, whereupon Molly joined in, which of course made them laugh even more. Then off she wandered back to the other caravan, where Sally found her later busily mixing up a mugful of milk, lemonade and washing up liquid. Maybe she was going to drink it; I don't know. She certainly wasn't going to wash dishes with it.

One day, while Sally and I were in the caravan lounge, Molly was standing at the sink in the caravan kitchen, happily sloshing cups and saucers around in lukewarm water, with not a bubble in sight. "I haven't been in here for a long time," she remarked, albeit untruthfully. "That's why I am so silly." I laughed out loud. "Oh, now we know, then!" and she chuckled. Sometimes, however, it is difficult to remain sunny while someone is doing a job that you know you will have to do all over again, and Sally exchanged glances with me and raised her eyes heavenwards. Walking over to Molly, she asked, "Don't you think it would be a good idea to use some washing-up liquid?"

"No thank you," replied Molly firmly, and there was no point in arguing. Half a minute later I went over to the sink and picked up the bottle. Squirting a good dollop into the bowl of water, I said, "There you go, that'll help you."

"Oh, thank you," replied Molly. There was never any point in reasoning with her or asking questions. If I so much as asked her which cake she would like, she could not decide, and we had constantly to remember that dementia was not just loss of memory, but of reasoning power and decision making. In short, a loss of brain cells.

Occasionally it also meant a loss of Molly's recent sunny nature, and a return to the elderly lady who could be awkward, stubborn and unco-operative. Bath-time was a case in point. All suggestions of ablutions would be greeted with a scowl, and even if I managed to coax and cajole her into undressing and standing in the water, *no way* was she going to sit down. Sometimes I was so exasperated that I got the shower attachment and gave her an all over gentle spray, but she would protest all the time, and of course this method did not reach the parts that mattered - which is why I tried to get her to sit down. So I gave up. At least her clothes were clean.

Sometimes even a change of clothes was a struggle. Finding her downstairs one morning, kneeling on the floor to clean the carpet by hand, I launched into porky-pie mode.

"Hi Molly! I've got some new trousers for you!"

"Oh have you?" she replied disinterestedly, continuing to pick up bits of dust and fluff.

"Yes, they're upstairs. Shall we go up and try them on?

"If you must."

"Come on then. We'll see if they fit." And up we trudged. The trousers weren't new, and she didn't know that, but she objected anyway.

"Well, I don't like these! Look, they've got ... all these things on!" and she plucked at some pulled threads, scowling. So I got out another pair, plus clean undies and blouse, and eventually managed the entire ensemble to the background of grumbles: It's too hot; it's too cold; I liked *those*; I don't like these; this is silly; why...? etc. She did admit, though, that her knickers were a bit grubby - with skid marks like Brands Hatch race track, she could hardly say otherwise.

I still managed to cut her hair occasionally, but she regarded the process with just a little less aversion than a bath. A session might go something like this:

Jane: "Your hair needs a little trim. Shall I give you a haircut?"

Molly: "No, not really."

Jane, who doesn't do taking No for an answer: "Oh, but I've come over specially to do it for you."

Molly: "Have you really?"

Jane: "Yes. It won't take long; shall we ...". I wheedled, leading her into the bathroom, and eventually got her head over the bath. I then applied some apparently horrible shampoo...

"I don't like *that*"!

...and water the wrong temperature. "Is that too hot ...?"

"Yes!"

"... or cold?"

"Yes!"

Constant moans of don't-do-that, and I-*said*-don't-do-that followed, and when I gave her a towel she started rubbing her head so hard with it that I had to tell her to leave some hair on. When I wielded the scissors there were still more moans, so I asked if she was in a bad mood.

"Yes."

"Why?"

"I always am."

"No, you're not. You're usually quite sunny. Anyway, I'm not scared of you. You can be as foul tempered as you like."

Silence. Maybe she'd like a drink? I offered her a glass of cranberry juice, which she drank as though it were going out of fashion. Then she pushed the glass away. "I don't like it. I hate it." It was seldom sufficient these days to utter the first statement; the following was always added for emphasis.

* * * * *

Fortunately such bad moods were rare, but there was a worse problem that summer. Molly started having a few problems with her potty training, specifically Number Two's. One day, Sally left her in the caravan lounge while she herself went to the loo and when she came out a few minutes later her nostrils were violently assaulted. It took only seconds for her nose to lead her to a Tupperware jug which had been used for the purpose and then put back onto the draining board. Molly must have known that she had done wrong, for she had completely disappeared from the scene of crime. The next time it happened, she used Martin's muesli bowl, and again she had scarpered. Both jug and bowl got slung into the bin. Bleach might well remove the germs, but not the memory.

Sally could just about cope with this, but more scary tales came from across the pond.

The latest caper is Pob going to have a quick pee, so quick in fact that she doesn't pull her pants down all the way and ends up peeing into them. Then they get pulled up again and everything's ok, right? At home, Jill makes a point of going in the bog every time that Pob does, so everything's fine, but yesterday when she picked up Pob from "work", Jill noticed that her back was wet. Fortunately, there is a pack of bed liners in the car, so the upholstery was spared. Ironically, the bed liners don't seem to be necessary in her bed.............so far.

The difficult thing to remember was that the old ladies were not incontinent; nor were they being awkward. They were doing what made sense to them at the time. A slightly more pleasant example was Pob's emptying the dregs from the teapot into the waste paper basket instead of down the sink. But Molly could top that one. For reasons known only to herself at the time, she completely blocked the washbasin in her upstairs bathroom by stuffing the plughole full of orange segments. Of course, once she had filled the basin, she couldn't empty it, so she did what anyone of sense would do and bailed it out. Various mugs and plant bowls were dotted all around the bathroom, full of dirty, stinking water, but the basin still wasn't empty. It took Martin and me to clear up the mess, he grovelling on the floor and wielding a large spanner, while I held a mug to collect what was left of the E-coli soup as he removed the u-bend. Double - no make that treble - yeeeeeeeeeeeeeeeuk. I shan't tell you what it looked like as it gushed out, but I am sure you have a good imagination. It took half a bottle of bleach to get everything back to normal. Sally also hid the plug, in case Molly left the water running, but, bearing in mind how well Molly could improvise, this was a pretty futile gesture.

When we related the tale to Norma, she suggested we ask Amie if she could get Molly a weekly away-day at Morwenna Residential Home, our nearest care home, where they would be able to give her a bath. So once again we contacted Amie, who agreed to try, but also made two very salient points to put our minds at rest: one, who would want to take off their clothes when they were comfortable and warm? two, a bath isn't that important. Bearing in mind that Molly probably went at least a year without one before I started on her the previous October, and that she rarely smelled, Amie was probably right.

As the Morwenna visits would take a few weeks to sort out, I made one more valiant attempt as lady's maid. Well, *I* think I was valiant. I breezed into the bungalow one morning and said firmly, "OK, Molly, you can have a bath, a hair-wash or both. Which would you like?"

"Neither," she replied immediately. No change there, then; on to Plan B. I went into the bathroom, ran the water with the shower attachment and said, "Hey, come in here a minute, Molly and feel this." She did so. "Kneel down, it will be easier." She did. "I'll just tuck this towel round your neck and it will be better. Just hold it there." She did. "Now is that too hot?" And her hair got washed.

Further cajoling resulted in her sitting sedately on a chair while I cut and blow dried her hair again - chopping off at least three inches in case it was another three months until I succeeded again.

"There," I said. "You *do* look beautiful!"

"Oh blimey!" she cackled, but seemed pleased. Half an hour later, when we were in the car, I put down her sun visor and she caught sight of herself in the mirror. Seizing the opportunity for further self congratulation, I said, "Your hair looks good, doesn't it?"

"No, I don't like it."

"Oh! I thought it looked really nice."

"Well, I don't like it, I hate it!"

This had now became a catch phrase in the family and seldom failed to produce a smile. I drove on.

* * * * *

Life with Molly contained constant surprises. We were becoming so used to her naughtiness that a successful summer visit from the travelling chiropodist had us slack-jawed with incredulity. We sat Molly in the sherb, a plate of food on her lap, and hoped she would not be too obstructive, but she behaved herself impeccably, giggling if he inadvertently tickled her feet, and sticking her fingers in her ears when he used the electric toenail-grinder. She even thanked him and asked, "How much should I give you?" I believe he, remembering her past performance, was as amazed as we were.

Two days later, Sally went up to Molly's bedroom with a plate of supper and walked into a snowstorm. The floor, chairs, dressing table and bed were covered with pieces of something resembling cotton wool, large chunks thrown haphazardly onto the floor or wedged into crevices, smaller pieces floating into the air again as Sally walked past. Shaking her head, Sally ignored the mess for a moment and took the food to Molly who was sitting on the bed oblivious to the chaos. Molly took the plate of food and said, "Right, I'm going home now." Sally, having learned not to contradict, used diversionary tactics and said, "Wouldn't you rather get into bed? It's much warmer there. Where's your rabbit?" Rabbit was a huge, white stuffed bunny sent to Molly by Heather from Canada, and it usually spent the night in bed with her. Sally looked round for it, and there it was, sitting on a chair with its head lolling over its shrunken, un-stuffed body. Molly the Ripper had struck again.

The trail of destruction continued. We found books with whole pages cut out of them; photograph albums emptied of their contents; photo frames with no pictures. Jewellery was picked apart, jigsaw puzzle pieces were stuffed into cups half full of cold tea. Toilet paper was torn off the roll, screwed into little balls and left everywhere. Tapes were removed from cassettes, the patchwork quilt was picked to pieces and anything that could be taken apart, was. From earlier years when Molly would arrange anything from flowers to cheese biscuits, she now seemed to want to de-range them. And no pun is intended. She may have had her reasons, if not her reason, but we couldn't fathom it, so just had to be careful to keep important things out of her reach. We failed, often.

Martin was in the caravan kitchen one morning when he heard a strange noise from the lounge. Looking across, he beheld Molly sitting on the sofa with one of Sally's tea towels, carefully cutting it in half with the bread saw. Martin remonstrated in his gentle way, "I don't think you should be doing that, Molly!" to which she replied crossly, still wielding the knife, "Well, it wasn't me!"

When Sally asked Molly later why she had done it, Molly pointed to one half of the tea towel and said, "Well, that's *that* ..." looked at the other half and was silent.

"What's *that*, then?" Sally asked.

"*I* don't know!" replied Molly with one of her shrug-flounces, and walked off.

Neither did we, and that just about summed up the whole situation.

CHAPTER 19

SAINTS ALIVE

Meanwhile, what of our friends in America? It had been a while since I heard from them, but this was eventually explained by the following email, very un-pc but very Adrian!

Our server went down recently, so I was doomed to spend hours on the phone with technical support, which is outsourced to India. That really was an experience. Talk about the "wisdom of the East" - it was more like talking to Peter Sellers. "Goodness gracious me, I really am sorry for all your trouble, I must put you on hold for a few minutes while I go outside and see to my elephant. He is shitting all over the place, you see, goodness gracious me..." Anyway, it is sorted out now, but no thanks to those buggers in Bangalore.

So Adrian and I continued to send irregular news of our respective mothers (in law), providing a deal of mutual support, and some smiles too. From Adrian:

We have learned that ice cream, which Pob loves, must be bought in a tub, not in a package, because there is no guarantee that it is going to be put back in the freezer. I have just hidden the stainless steel scourer, as she was about to start on a Tefal pan. A couple of days ago, Jill gave her the job of cooking a couple of corn cobs, and Pob tried to bake them in the oven at 450 degrees F in a PLASTIC dish. The inside of the oven looked as though the gob monster from the planet goo had invaded. The pity is that Pob knew she had buggered it up, but had absolutely no idea why or how.

I breathed another sigh of relief that Molly had given up cooking so long ago, not attempting to make so much as a cup of tea nowadays. Pob, however, ploughed valiantly on.

Yesterday we had another first. In spite of our resolve to make all the cuppas ourselves, she found the kettle and tried to make tea without putting any water in it. She couldn't make out why it never boiled. Fortunately, it has over-heat protection on it. As for real drinks, she always enjoyed a gin and tonic, but now she could be given anything, lemonade even, and wouldn't know the difference. Furthermore, alcohol seems to have little effect on her. We left her alone for about an hour last Saturday morning, and when we got back she said she had made herself a cup of coffee, and was drinking something out of a coffee mug. But it wasn't coffee, it was rum, and she had drunk a mugful of it at least, judging from the drop in level in the rum bottle. About ten minutes later she passed out, and slept for six hours. Then she recovered, apparently none the worse for the experience, dammit.

I could well understand Adrian's seemingly brutal, but actually just honest, mindset with regard to his mother-in-law, but I was really sorry when he told me that Jill was frequently reduced to tears over Pob. In a way, we were mourning the loss of our mothers already, but sometimes Molly seemed so normal that it was hard to believe anything was wrong. But AD is like a fungus; what you find on the surface appears only after the underground network has spread and taken hold. Then the mushrooms just keep popping up all the time. We would find the bread and butter in the drawer, Christmas decorations in the bathroom in May, another pair of knickers (thankfully, clean) in the fridge and nasty little surprises in kitchenware.

Jill and Adrian's worst problem was that they had moved out of their own house to live with Pob, which meant that they could not send Pob back home at night. Pob went to her "job" for seven hours a day, when Adrian was at home, but this was no help to Jill who was out at work all day. Relief came in the spring when Jill took some time off.

I just cannot describe how great it is for the two of us to have some time alone while Pob is "at work", wrote Adrian. *We can both be more patient with her when we have seven hours a day to de-frazzle. Incidentally, Pob, because she is still with it enough to know that she isn't paid, commented that it didn't seem to be much of a job if it didn't yield a pay cheque...........so, guess what? I had a word with "the boss", and now, lo! every Friday she gets a cheque for $250.00, and she is happy as hell.*

The cheque was, of course, unsigned or otherwise un-useable, but it kept Pob happy, and in spite of his frequent protestations of being hard-hearted, and his Dammit remark when Pob survived her binge drinking, I think this salary episode demonstrated what a caring person Adrian was. He was even perturbed about this little gem:

Jill takes Pob out shopping sometimes and walks her around the mall until she is exhausted, and then we can leave her for an hour or two, knowing that she's too tired to get up to anything. Christ, forgive us, for we are very cruel.

I did not share Adrian's opinion. I thought he and Jill were saints. But lots of people told Sally and me that we were too, and we never thought of ourselves as such. No, let me correct that. I thought of Sally as one.

It was now early summer, and Molly had changed into lighter clothes. She seemed to have little sense, however, of the actual temperature, for she would wear just as many layers as she had done in mid-winter. I arrived one morning to find her in two jumpers and a jacket, and over everything a blue blouse. She had one arm through a sleeve and the rest of the blouse buttoned diagonally across her chest. I extricated her, made some lunch, and we ate together in the sherb. She picked at her food, and, although she said she was fine, did not seem quite herself, and was coughing frequently. Later, when I checked with Sally, I learned that Molly had not eaten her breakfast, and that Sally had made her a doctor's appointment for the next day. Molly was diagnosed with a chest infection and prescribed two weeks' worth of antibiotics. This meant yet more pills, and Sally walked away from the surgery with a sinking feeling.

To Bella's delight, for three weeks or more, Molly spent most days in bed, but even so was not really aware of how poorly she was. If we asked, "How are you today?" she would reply, "Fine." If we said, "You're looking better," she would ask, "What do you mean?" Then she had more dizzy spells, which alarmed us so much that we called the doctor again. His tests showed that it wasn't a TIA, or mini stroke, as we had feared, rather that the infection had spread to Molly's ears and was affecting her balance. Poor Molly was having a rough time.

Sally had an even rougher time, as a second dose of antibiotics was prescribed and she had to get Molly to swallow them. The trouble was, Molly tended to chew her tablets, and these were huge, the Scud missiles of the pill world, and tasted foul. Sally tried crushing them and mixing them in jam, but sometimes that too failed. One morning Molly refused even to take the spoon (as if she *remembered* it would taste nasty?) until eventually Sally pleaded, "Come on, Molly, do it for me. Make me happy." Molly took the spoon from her, and Sally smiled in relief, but the smile froze on her face as Molly flung the jam straight onto the floor. Exasperated beyond saintliness, Sally stomped off to Martin, sitting with a friend in his lounge.

"Uh-oh," remarked Martin, hearing the stomps and seeing Sally's face. "Looks like I'm in trouble."

"No," said Sally. "It's not you, it's Molly." She told her tale and got lots of sympathy, plus more from me later. That evening though, when I retold it to John, I saw the funny side and could hardly speak.

"That reminds me of when Angus was little," said John, when I had finally spluttered to the end. "He would sit in his high chair, put on that I'm-going-to-see-how-far-I-can-go grin, then pick up his big red spoon and lob spoonfuls of his dinner at the wall. And because of his cheeky face and the sheer naughtiness, we ended up laughing too - for the first couple of throws anyway."

Sally had not found Molly's naughtiness so funny, and, to give her a break, I said I would try to get the next Scud into Molly. I managed, by dint of cutting it into four, inserting each fragment into a small piece of chocolate-coated cereal bar, and pretending each one was something different:

"Here's a sweetie for you, Molly."

"Ooh, thank you." Munch, munch.

"Here's another. See if you like this kind better."

"Ooh, thank you."

"Here's a sweetie for you, Molly."

"Ooh..."

"How about this one?"

And so on.

I described the above to Adrian in yet another email, and his irreverent response had me laughing once more.

Pob takes a helluva lot of pills too, but her trick is just to use her mouth as a storage bin. If she is not told to swallow them, she won't. Not just with pills either. On barbecue evenings, when we grill up large chunks of some unfortunate bull's bum, we usually have some shrimp (prawns to you) as an appetiser. Pob will stick a shrimp in her mouth and chances are it will still be there half an hour later. Still, it's cheaper that way.

One way or another, we managed to get Molly to swallow her pills, and gradually the cure seemed to take effect and she was coughing less. We were now into the third week, though, which meant the third Tuesday running that I had not taken her with me on the shopping run, and I really missed her help. Plus I had other duties to do for her. She was now totally unable - or unwilling - to change her clothes, and one morning I found her lying on the bed wearing a pair of rather yucky knickers over her trousers. Moving Bella to the side of the bed, I took the opportunity to remove everything in Molly's nether regions, including an even yuckier pair of knickers under the trousers. At least it was easier tackling her lying down, or perhaps it was the fact that she was not feeling up to scratch that made her more biddable than usual. After I had put clean clothes on her, I put the dirty washing in a carrier bag, then noticed the bag had a tear in it.

"Oh dear," I said, holding it up to show Molly. "I shall have to get another one. Never mind, plenty of old bags round here!"

She laughed with me then, but as she got better and fitter, performing the weekly sartorial number on her became more of a struggle. Usually I managed the full ensemble, but one day I gave up having done only the bottom layer. When I got home, where we were having structural alterations made to the kitchen, our builder friend had been knocking seven bells out of the chimney, the place was covered in brick dust and soot, and he looked like I felt, worn out.

"Well, I bet you've been having more fun than I have," I told him.

"No," he puffed, "I'd rather be doing anything than this."

"OK, we'll swap then," I suggested.

"So, what have you been up to?"

"Getting Mother's knickers off."

"Phew!" he replied, looking quite frightened, "I think I'll stick to knocking down chimneys." I rather thought I might join him.

Molly continued to rally, and ventured outside again. Martin found her at the back door wearing Bella's blanket as a poncho, and struggling to get a welly boot on.

"Having trouble, Molly?" he enquired.

"I can't ...do ... this *thing*!" she replied, pushing at the boot ineffectually. Martin looked closer.

"Well, there's your problem! Let's get this off, shall we?" and he carefully removed a cushion cover from her foot.

"Thank you," she said politely, as though being divested of a cushion cover were an everyday occurrence, and continued on her journey up the garden path.

Sally found her back indoors later, sitting up in bed with a green rag across her knees - a runner bean costume worn by one of the girls in a carnival when they were little; heaven knows where she had found it. A cup of cold tea sat on the bedside table, a tissue in Molly's hand, and she was dipping the tissue in the tea and using it to wipe down the rag. Sally didn't say a word, just thought, Time to go! And went.

* * * * *

Sally and I always found our exchanges of amusing experiences immensely uplifting. We were not hurting Molly by laughing, and although we were only too aware of how sad the whole experience was, we knew that she too would have laughed, had it been her mother as the star of the show, and so would Smithy. Sometimes, like Adrian, I thought maybe I was being callous in not devoting more time to Molly, but there were so many other things to fit into my life. Most of the time we did spend together was quality time, and I would share the humorous side of the situation with her as often as I could.

Molly and I had always had a good relationship. I was a model child (OK, I'll pass you the bucket, but I was) and, as I grew older, she and I found shared interests, opinions, humour and general ways of doing things. People even called me Molly's carbon copy. With Sally, it was always different. As a child, Sally was charming, cute, bubbly and friendly. Everyone loved her - they still do. But she and Molly just didn't click. Also, Sally being the first child, Molly was strict with her, standing no nonsense and refusing many of her requests, even simple ones like bringing a friend round to tea. Sally reckons that she, big sister, paved the way for me, but, as I see it, I was better at sweet-talking my mother, not being naughty, and simply doing my own thing without asking permission.

During Sally's teens the relationship worsened. It was not until we all left home that things improved and the three of us became more like friends. Then, when Sally's first marriage broke up, Molly disowned her for two years. She would never have done that to me. I mention this because Sally, naturally, never forgot any of it, which I think makes her even more of a saint to look after Molly as she does. On the rare occasion when Sally *might* sense that she is treating Molly in a callous way, she can make herself feel better by remembering how Molly used to treat *her*.

Sally and I both did our best for Molly, and I believed that she had had a really good innings, especially as she was now approaching 80. We would continue to place her interests high on our agenda, but we were very much aware that our families merited first place in our lives; for my part especially the bit with John in it.

Which reminds me ... coming home after one of my bedtime battles with Molly's fashion show, I went in to wake John from an afternoon power nap in our bedroom, and found our Jo-Jo cat cuddled up to him, purring blissfully. I stood talking with him for a moment, then said, "Well, I had better go. I have things to do, and if I stand here, I might think you are Molly lying there with Bella and come and change your knickers for you." John smiled sleepily.

"Oh!" I added, turning to go. "You'd probably like that!"

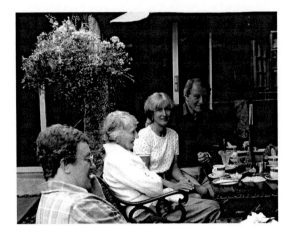

Cream Tea at Cadgwith.
2003
Norma, Molly, Jane, John

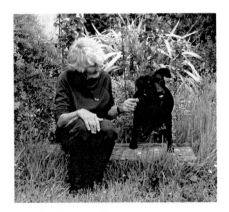

Molly and Tilly in Parc Bush
garden. Summer 2003

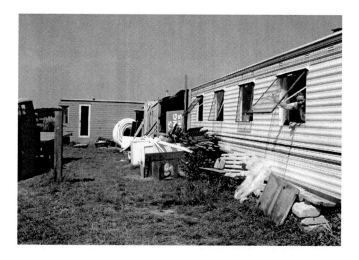

The Funny Farm. Summer 2004

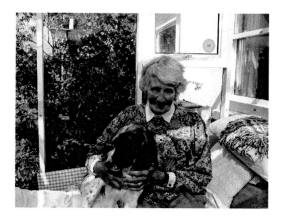

Molly and Clem in the "sherb"
Summer 2004

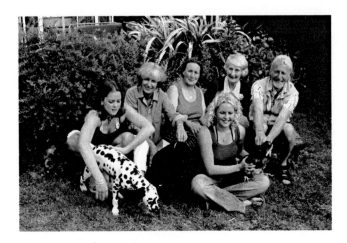

The Crazy Gang on
Molly's 80th birthday.
Toana, Bernard, Jane, Tilly,
Sally, Molly, Royce, Wenna and
chicken

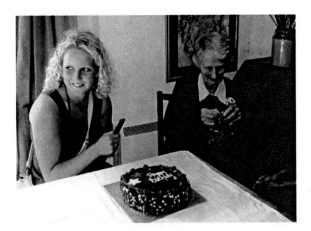

A rare moment: Molly ignoring
cake.

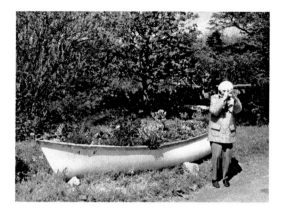

Prazegooth 2006
Same hat as first day at
school!

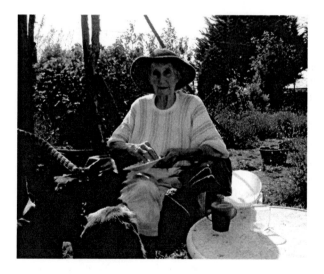

Molly today aged 83

CHAPTER 20

MIDSUMMER MADNESS

Although Molly's chest infection was fading, her prolonged stint in bed had done her no good at all physically. She had stiffened up so much that she even had difficulty getting downstairs. Some mornings she would lie in bed for hours. Sally did her best to get her up, because the more she lay in bed the stiffer she became, and one day she was cajoling Molly, saying, "You can't stay in bed all day."

"Well, what time is it?" asked Molly.

"Nearly one o' clock."

"Well, that's only half the day, isn't it?"

Sometimes the flashes of the old Molly were quite breathtaking. And how on earth was she able to remember that one o'clock was roughly the middle of the day, when so much else escaped her completely?

The stiffness, however, really was a problem. I was in the middle of breakfast at home one morning when I got a panic phone call from Sally. Molly was stuck in bed; could I come round?

I arrived at Parc Bush to find Sally and Wenna looking down helplessly on Molly as she lay on the bed in her dormer bedroom, clutching a cuddly toy seal and unable to move. She had managed to swing round a little, but was now stuck on her back diagonally with her head almost on the banisters and her legs in the wardrobe, dainty feet swollen and painful to such an extent that Sally thought one might be broken. Every time we tried to move her, she protested and started hyperventilating. So we propped her feet on a cushion and waited for the doctor, standing around like guests at a soirée, while Molly reclined happily, nursing her stuffed seal, staring at the ceiling and uttering inanities, all of which we concurred with.

Molly: "It's a stant."

Jane: "Yes, it sure is, but not to worry."

Molly: "Look at him up there!" pointing to the empty top of the wardrobe.

Wenna: "Oh goodness, yes! I wonder what he's up to!"

Molly: "I haven't got two drovs to niv."

Sally: "I know. Nor have I!"

And more of same. It is amazingly easy to have these worthless exchanges once you get used to it, which might sound patronising, but how else do you deal with it? Besides, really, how worthy are our own conversations, blethering on about the weather, gossip and ... just stuff? Nothing earth-shattering, is it? Much of it is no more than the human equivalent of monkeys picking fleas off each other, only not so useful.

The doctor came in double quick time, checked that nothing was broken, and then patiently coaxed Molly to stand up. This took about fifteen minutes but eventually she made it. Wenna was an absolute star. She jollied Molly along, made her laugh, helped her get up and walk to the bathroom, and made no fuss at all about aiding her gran to get trousers and drawers off, sit on the loo - all of which took another ten minutes - and cheer when the sound of tinkles was heard. Soon after that, Molly was able to walk across to the caravan and take up her usual position on one of the sofas. "I'm going to sit on my plang," she said with a smile. She then ate her breakfast and carried on as though nothing untoward had happened; which, as far as she would remember, it hadn't.

* * * * *

The summer was building up to Sally's busy time at The Crow's Nest, her craft shop in the local village, so I offered to see to Molly one morning soon after the above story. Molly was lying in bed when I arrived, Bella in her usual position on the patchwork quilt alternately purring contentedly and hissing at the dogs. I wasn't sure that Molly would be keen to climb out of bed, so this was my first problem, best tackled with a bright and breezy "nursey" tone, stopping just short of addressing Molly in the first person plural.

"Coo-ee!" I shrieked as I walked upstairs.

"Who's that?" from the bed.

"It's me!"

Perhaps I should explain here that Molly seldom used our Christian names when she was pre-AD, and afterwards the seldom became less and less. As I said earlier, she had never addressed John by his name, and by now it would be difficult to say whether she would recognise any of ours. Voices, however, like faces, were a different matter, and she knew it was me shouting up the stairs as soon as she heard me.

"Oh hello," she said, as I hove into view.

"I'm going shopping," I announced. "Want to come?" This temptation usually worked.

"Yes, OK. What do I have to do?"

"Well, get yourself out of bed, and we'll get ready."

This sometimes took a few minutes, while Molly gingerly slid herself off the mattress, but that day she was relatively sprightly. Dressing was no problem, as she slept fully clothed, but her ancient navy cardigan with huge red buttons did look rather scruffy. Since she seemed in a good mood, I thought I would chance a change.

"What about a nice green cardigan to go with your blouse?" I enquired. The blouse was yellow, but so what?

"Yes, all right," and I managed to divest her of the navy monstrosity before she changed her mind, and get her into a pretty, pale green one. Molly's dormer bedroom opens out straight from the stairs, which can be very handy at times, and the blue thing was chucked over the banisters on its way to the wash, possibly the dustbin, without her even noticing. While my luck held, I ventured a change of footwear. "Which socks shall we have - this nice stripey pair, or some plain ones?"

Molly could not actually make such a decision, and I knew this full well, but it gave her the power of the moment in expressing her opinion as to *which* socks, rather than asking her did she *want* a clean pair and risking her (almost certain) reply of "No."

She replied as I had hoped, "Oh, I don't mind," and the stripes it was. Suggesting she sit down, I took off her sandals (she had slept in those too) and pink socks within seconds, and encased her feet in green, orange and yellow lurex stripes without her even flinching.

Next the loo. Sally and I knew, from dropping toilet paper down the pan occasionally, that Molly did use and flush the loo, so I suggested to her that she might like to go. I wasn't sure how to phrase it; would the old fashioned version "go to the toilet" make a better connection that "use the loo" or "have a wee"? I risked the former.

"Where?" she asked, and I pointed her in the direction of the en suite. Off she went, coming out again three seconds later.

"With this?" she asked, proffering a long piece of toilet roll that she had torn off.

One must always remember with AD not to be negative, so I replied, "Yes, that's right. Now, do you want to use the loo?" just in case she had not understood "go to the toilet". Back she went. Not wanting to invade her privacy, I did not follow her in, just listened. "I don't know what to do," she muttered. Oh God! I would have to go in. Then I found that if I stood in a certain place I could catch her reflection in the glass panel of the open door, see that she was sitting down, trousers and knickers round ankles as required, and hear the appropriate noises. Obviously she was still fully able to use the toilet, but just had not understood when someone asked her to. She adjusted her clothes properly and tried to flush the loo. At that point I went in to help her, suggesting that she push the lever a bit harder, which she duly did. I was then able to further suggest that she wash her hands at the basin, an unusual procedure these days. She did this properly, using soap and towel, and we were ready to go downstairs and walk across to the caravans for breakfast.

Breakfast comprised toast and marmalade, a drink and, most important of all, The Pills. Molly had been quite good, for most of the last five years, at taking the wretched things, the only problem being, at first, that she forgot them. We had tried everything, starting with little jars marked with the days of the week, but these had never worked because Molly never knew what day it was. Then we bought her a clock that told her the days, but she insisted on keeping this in the lounge, while her pills were in the kitchen. Finally, Sally and I found it was easier and more reliable to administer the pills ourselves. This had worked for ages, and Molly would usually swallow them immediately. If she did object, or try to tell us she had already had them, we would say OK, leave it for half a minute and start again. By which time she had forgotten the first attempt and would, nine times out of ten, take them like a lamb.

However, since the Scud missile version was added to the list, she seemed to remember (yes, really!) that pills were not nice. We were successful for a while with dismantling a piece of cake or a yoghurt raisin, stuffing the pill in there, and squidging it all together again, but even then we seldom completed the course, falling at the third or fourth tablet. So now we had taken to crushing the pills, mixing them in butter, spreading the mix on toast and smothering the whole slice in marmalade. The piece of toast was then cut into little pieces which were fed to her one at a time, making sure the dogs were out of the way. It was a painstaking process, but it worked.

Until this particular day. I had forgotten all about Tilly until I heard Molly whisper craftily, "I'll give you some in a minute," and I turned, too late, to see Tilly's jaws gratefully closing round a piece of toast, butter, marmalade and pills. That should sort *her* blood pressure out for the rest of the day. Tilly then got thrown outside, and so did Sally's dog Clem.

By now I had been at Parc Bush for an hour. But there was still the drink to be taken. Too impatient to make tea or coffee, I gave Molly some organic fruit juice, which today she enjoyed, followed by a bowl of summer fruits which she greeted with, "Urgh, I don't like this," and then tucked into with enthusiasm. This entailed a further ten minutes, while my fingers started to twitch and drum on the worktop. I admit it, I am not the most patient of souls, and would have made a hopeless nurse. Wondering how on earth Sally coped, then reflecting that at least she lived here and could get on with her life while she waited for Molly, I witnessed the final scraping of the dish, and reminded Molly of our day's mission.

"I'm going to Mullion. Would you like to come?"

"Ooh yes, all right then. Now?"

"Yes,"

"With you?"

"Yes, off we go,"

"Shall I ...?"

"Yes, you come along with me," and off we went to the car.

"Ooh, are we going in this?" she asked.

"Yes, in you pop."

"What, here?"

"Yes, you hop in ..." in she got and I handed her the seat belt ... "and put that in the red thing."

Then I walked round to the other side of the car, got into the driver's seat, and prepared to remove her seat belt from my clip. Heavens! There was no need.

"Crikey, you've put it in the right one for a change!" I exclaimed, and she laughed with glee.

Off we went. We passed Winnie and Albert's house next door and I decided to test her memory. "Do you remember Winnie and Albert?" I asked.

Molly reflected for a second. "No, not really."

"Well, they used to live next door to you, but Winnie died a little while ago."

I held my breath to see if there was any reaction.

"Oh! What a shame!" and I could tell by her tone that she had fully taken in the seriousness of what I had told her. It is too easy to think that because AD sufferers have trouble expressing themselves, they cannot understand what they hear. Very often, they can. I changed to more cheerful subjects, and soon Molly was making her own contributions, exclaiming at how wiggly the road was, and trying to read the road signs.

We duly arrived at Mullion and, while I popped into the chemist, she elected to stay in the car, which was fine - she had never yet tried to escape from it. Then we went to the Post Office and chose three cards for her forthcoming 80th birthday. I knew she would enjoy looking at them, and she chuckled at quite a few; not the ones that were meant to be funny - they went right over her head - but little quirky things, like odd shaped flowers and animals, and one in particular that repeated "Smile" about two dozen times. "Look," she said, pointing at the line of words, "it says S-S-S- ..." - she couldn't quite say it.

"Better do what it says, then!" I said, and she laughed again.

I picked out an "I am 80" badge, and got her to read it aloud. "That will be you in three weeks' time," I told her.

"Oh will it?"

"Yes, isn't it amazing? Do you like this card?" and I showed her one with a picture of a squirrel on it, plus the words, "You Are What You Eat". Inside it said "Nuts". She loved the squirrel, so I bought the card.

Eventually we ambled up to the counter, where she was solicitous that I paid for my handbag as well as for the cards, and we came back to Parc Bush. Taking her into her lounge, I showed her a jig saw puzzle in pieces on the table.

"Have you seen this?" I asked. Even her failing memory had registered that she had done it something approaching 50 million times since Christmas, but with an eager "Ooh yes!" she homed in on it and started fitting the pieces together. It was a twenty piece puzzle for 5-7 year olds and she probably had more pleasure from that small, simple thing than anything else in the past year. I left her happily jig-sawing and went home.

* * * * *

When I told Molly again, on 26 August, that she was 80, she was very surprised. I made sure she wore her "I am 80" badge, so that we could point to it and remind her every so often, and we held a party to mark the occasion. If she was surprised at that too, she didn't show it. Because her birthday was, as usual, on a bank holiday weekend (how did Nan manage to find a maternity hospital with staff on duty? It wouldn't happen these days!), many invitees were, sadly, not able to come, although all sent special greetings. Norma and Dudley were alone among Molly's friends to manage to get there, but family and our own friends swelled the ranks, and somehow Sally and I found the time to organise the whole event. Did I say organise? Well, we muddled through it somehow. We garnered enough food to feed however many cohorts turned up, then turned our attentions to Parc Bush. This mostly involved flinging everything that was on a table or worktop into a cupboard, vacuuming a week's (OK, several months') dust, and making sure there were enough chairs for all the bottoms likely to arrive.

It was a case of all hands on deck, even the men. John took the opportunity to put up some banister rails for Molly, something he had been meaning to do for months, so she could now hang on to a rail from the bottom of the stairs all the way up, through the bedroom and right along to the loo. Martin went down the garden with spade and wheelbarrow, bringing back a precarious barrowload of lettuce, tomatoes, beetroot, potatoes, carrots and herbs; every single vegetable and salad item on the table came from his veggie patch. He even made a carrot and beetroot cake. The table was filled with food, the freezer stuffed with bottles to quick-chill beer and white wine; paper crockery and cups were arranged and we awaited the first guest.

Sally and I had great plans for Molly, namely bath, hair wash and best party frock, but, after a couple of failed attempts, we wisely abandoned these in favour of a token gesture with the facecloth, some clean trousers and a pretty top, and handing her the hairbrush while she ate breakfast. Any suggestion that she might actually like to *use* the brush was met with resistance and the likelihood of the brush being thrown across the room, so we dropped that idea too in the pursuance of peace.

First to arrive were Royce and Patti, always a treat as we saw so little of them. They had zoomed over from Bodinnick on Royce's motorbike, and we just had time to catch up on a little family news, when Molly, having walked over from the caravan, arrived at the door.

"Come in, Mother!" I cried. "Royce and Patti are here!"

"Who?" asked Molly.

"Royce. Your son."

"I don't know," she answered. "Oh all right," and she came in and said a polite hello to what she saw as two strangers. Followed by several more.

Our next guests were our good friends Tess and John Barlow, with daughter Anna who had just majored in pottery and ceramics. She had turned her artistic flair in the direction of birthday cup-cakes for Molly, and you have never seen anything like it. Myriad colours in royal icing, swirls, twirls, cherries, blobs, dots, rosettes and stripes, the perfect gift for one who adores not only cake but pretty colours and patterns too. Molly was delighted, and continued to be for the next three days, each time we gave her a cake being like the first.

After that, people arrived in droves, and I scarcely had time to slosh a drink into a cup for them and speak half a sentence, before it was time to do the same for the next - and of course grab a bite to eat myself. What do you mean, *and some alcohol?* I had been doing that since 11.00 a.m.!

Molly was having a ball. She had cards, flowers, chocolates, cakes, teddy bears, socks, and even a phone call from Auntie Heather in Canada - all delightfully received and appreciated. Everything went swimmingly for some hours, right up to cake cutting time, but by then Molly was a little tired and crotchety. That is the p.c. interpretation. The uncharitable among us would have said the attention had gone to her head and she was behaving like a spoiled brat. When we placed her specially gooey chocolate cake in front of her and gave her a knife, she ignored both and focused all her attention on the wet tablecloth. Someone had spilled wine on it and, no matter how much we said it didn't matter, she obviously thought it did. She continued to poke it, pull it, peer at it and all but pick it up and launder it. Eventually I folded the wet corner back under the rest of the cloth, and redirected her attention to the cake. To make it easier, we had already put the knife in, as it were.

"Look, Molly," I said, pointing to the implement, "just press the knife down. OK?"

Molly ignored me. Wenna came to help, and she can be charm itself when she chooses. Sitting beside her gran, she wheedled to the best of her ability. "Come on Molly, just cut the cake. Do it for me!"

All we got were shakings of her head and downright refusals. "Norma," I said to our friend who was sitting close by with an I've-seen-it-all-before expression, "you're the expert, would you like to try?"

"No, thank you," she said, with a firm shake of her head. Who could blame her? Time for some humour.

"You are an awkward old bat, Mother, aren't you?" I said mildly. "Just push the knife down. It's really easy."

"All right," said the old bat, and her wicked sense of humour surfaced once more as, with a sudden swipe of her hand, she knocked the knife away from her, sending it and chocolate gloop flying across the table. And, as most mischievous children do, Molly got her reaction; a round of laughter.

The cake was delicious, in spite (or because) of being stuffed full of E-numbers and hydrogenated vegetable oil, and we did full justice to it. Then Patti called all the Smiths into the garden to have our photos taken beside the pond. In spite of having to sit there for several minutes, squinting at the sun until we almost went blind, the results weren't bad. Even a couple of dogs and a chicken got in on the act. Then Royce offered to take me for a spin on his 800+cc motorbike to The Lizard and back. Potentially scary as this was, I had implicit faith in his driving abilities, so instead it was just exhilarating.

People began to drift off just as we got back, but a good time was had by all, especially the birthday girl, and it would be one to remember. We were thankful that so many people thought of her. The old Molly would have been touched, as were we, her family.

* * * * *

An American birthday was being celebrated at about the same time and, although Pob was even less aware of the occasion than Molly, she too was in for a treat.

> Jill and two of her friends took Pob out to lunch (the expression "out to lunch" being exquisitely appropriate in the present circumstances) and it seems they had a very long merry meal. This morning Pob had forgotten everything, but Jill was very pleased with the way the day worked out and that, ironically, is the most important thing. Jill did it for herself, rather than for her mother, because she didn't want the old girl's birthday to pass unrecognised.

The fact that Jill did the lunch for herself rather than for Pob seemed eminently human and unremarkable to us. Although one does everything one can for the Pobs and Mols, one has to revert to being selfish (for want of a better word) because there is just no other way to get through it, and because the P/M's only know what is going on for a nanosecond. Sometimes it makes us think we are being hard, whereas in reality we are just surviving as best we can. No-one should have to go through all this, patient or carer, but we do, so no-one is going to blame us if we take to drink/laughter/religion or any other support. When it came to Jill's own birthday, Adrian had this to say:

> *Jill's birthday is coming up next week, and she mentioned this to Pob yesterday. When Pob seemed surprised, Jill asked her when she (Pob) thought her (Jill's) birthday was. The old girl had no clue, of course, even when cued, and finally Jill said in exasperation, "I don't understand why you don't know when my birthday is. You were there when I was born!"*
>
> *"Oh, was I?" was the reply.*

CHAPTER 21

THE LONGEST WEEKEND

Following Norma's suggestion, Amie, our CPN, succeeded fairly swiftly in arranging a weekly day-visit for Molly to Morwenna Residential Home, which was very handy, being just up the road from us at The Lizard. Morwenna was where Nan had spent her last days, and although she had hated it, she would have hated anything that wasn't her home, including Buckingham Palace. Molly's visits to Morwenna were different, arriving after breakfast, having lunch and tea, and being brought home again in the early evening. She enjoyed new and stimulating surroundings, chatting to all and sundry, wandering through the rooms at will, and taking with her any of her own bits and pieces she wanted. The Morwenna staff were kind and understanding, and, most important, willing. If they had time, and Molly was co-operative, they also gave her a bath. Whether Molly enjoyed her ride on the hoist to get in and out I am not sure, but it certainly made the job easier, and it was such a relief for Sally or myself when we collected Molly in the evening, all freshly washed and clad in clean clothes. All we had to do was deliver Molly and her clothes, bring her and her laundry home and pay £2 to cover her lunch. The local council funded the visits, and whatever else they and the state did not do, we were extremely grateful for this, and Sally could look forward to her break every week.

The strain of coping with Molly for the remaining six days, however, as well as managing her own life, did tell on Sally at times. So, when Royce and Patti offered to take her to The Isles of Scilly with their family for a long weekend, all expenses paid, she grabbed the chance and a suitcase, scraped together a small g&t fund, and flitted. Jolly good luck to her. She had earned a holiday, and four days didn't begin to recompense her for her endeavours with Molly, let alone life in general.

The trouble was, of course, that Sally was the Parc Bush C.O. and so her troops would be left to do battle all on their own. She and I had had several debates about how best to deal with Molly during Sally's Scilly holiday, and eventually we invited Social Services to come and put their oar in. This was not before time, but if you don't ask - which we hadn't - you don't get. A nice young man called Clive visited us at Parc Bush and did a thorough job of taking copious notes and asking questions about Molly. What was her date of birth? What did she eat? Could she dress herself? Did she have any particular hobby? Did she have a good memory?

Sally and I were speechless for several seconds before I said, "*Hello?* She is in the advanced stages of Alzheimer's!" No-one had told him, and apparently it was not on a file anywhere, which is pretty amazing considering all the other personal data that is available out there for all and sundry to make use of. Once we had got over this little misunderstanding, Clive was actually very helpful. As all the Morwenna beds were full for that particular weekend, he suggested respite care at The Gables in Redruth. We had heard good reports of this home from Norma, so, although it would involve us driving Molly there and bringing her home - a round trip each time of fifty miles - plus a fee worthy of a three star hotel, we thought it would be worth it.

Why, you might ask, were we so eager to farm Molly out while Sally was away? Why couldn't Martin, the girls and I manage? Quite simply, it was on account of the ponies (rhyming slang, *pony and trap* - work it out!). Sally had kept the muesli bowl episode from Martin and the girls for some time, but had to break it to them eventually. Fortunately, when she did, they thought it was so hysterically funny that it worked as a very good introduction to geriatric toilet habits. Recently, though, Molly had started leaving the little packets all over the house - deposited on work tops, smeared on cushions or hidden in drawers; sometimes gift wrapped in toilet paper or - of all things - a banana skin, sometimes *au naturel*.

The happy productions took place when Molly was left alone, but we were not sure why. Did she forget where the loo was? In the caravan this would be understandable, but not in her own home. Did she get caught short, not make it to the loo in time? But she never had trouble with "number ones", and was not actually incontinent. Was diet to blame? We knew there were some foods, lettuce for instance, that would give her Delhi belly. But, without getting too texturally explicit, Delhi didn't apparently come into it; and we thanked Ganesh and all the other Hindu gods for that small mercy at least.

The oddest thing was that on the one occasion when Sally tried to forestall the problem by showing Molly the loo and asking if she would like to use it, Molly replied, "What, *there*? Ugh, no thank you!"

What to do? We didn't believe that this problem alone made Molly sufficiently *non compos mentis* to have to live in a residential home. So, all one could say was ... shit happens; deal with it. Sally, however, was the only one sufficiently stalwart to do so. Because she had raised two children, it was no real problem to her, and once the initial Urgh was over, she took a deep breath (well, not too deep) and got on with the clearing up.

I couldn't do it. Were a cat or dog involved, I would be ... not *happy* exactly ... to clear it up, but not completely nauseated either. But human stuff? No way. Martin, Wenna and Toana felt the same. So, in the absence of Sally, we needed some other willing person, and a better paid one was the only solution.

So, there we were, Sally and I, sitting chatting to Clive, having almost decided that The Gables it would have to be, whatever the cost, when I happened to ask about a Care Package, which had been mentioned to us by Amie some years back. This is where a private care home, such as Polgoose in Helston, would send out someone on a daily basis to see to a patient's needs. We could not afford it then, but now we were eligible for some funding from Social Services.

"So would this be possible for a few days?" I asked Clive.

"Yes, we can arrange that," he replied, and I almost asked *Well, why didn't you suggest it?* but thought better of it.

"Great!" said Sally. "So Molly can stay at home and we shan't have to drive her to Redruth and back."

"What about the, er, little parcels?" I asked tentatively. "Will the care assistants be able to handle that? Sorry, I mean ..."

"I know what you mean," smiled Clive, "and yes, don't worry. They've seen everything."

So we settled on this solution. We felt it would be better for Molly at that stage not to have to leave home; plus it would be cheaper and would give us an introduction to the care that was available. Clive turned his attention to the forms in triplicate.

That night, Sally had another idea that came to her, she said, from a dream, and was so brilliant that it woke her up. What if Morwenna staff were prepared to take Molly during each day, even though they had no beds for a night-time stay? Then Martin and the girls would not have to worry about Molly at all, apart from taking her there and bringing her back at night. A quick phone call to Morwenna established a Yes to that too.

"So why," I asked Sally the next day when she told me of this, "did no-one suggest that to us either?"

"I don't know," replied Sally. "Seems we have to do all the thinking for ourselves, and it doesn't bloody help much when we're stressed out with that problem and several others at the same time."

I could only agree.

So everything was set up. Sally flew off west, and our ranks were temporarily swelled by Ellen, a private nurse from Polgoose. Ellen came out every day to "do" Albert, next door to Molly, and Martin's dad down the road, so it was no great trouble for her to pop in to Molly's afterwards to get her up, washed and dressed. Was it?

The first morning I got to Molly's just after ten o' clock to find that Ellen had already got Molly out of bed. So far so good. Then Ellen had sat her on the loo, knickers round ankles, and was running the hot water to wash her. First problem - no hot water. The immersion heater hadn't worked. It never rains, does it?

So I boiled a kettle and stood in the doorway to watch a professional do her job. Ellen was indeed professional, and efficient too. But ... I hate to say this ... she was in a rush and I don't think she was patient or kind. It seemed to me that she was used to treating wrinklies who had all their faculties and could be jollied along, and if they were told to do this and that, they would do it. But AD is such a different proposition. Plus Molly was dressed only in her bra and blouse and was complaining of the cold.

"Do you want the heater on?" I asked Ellen, meaning Is Molly Cold? But Ellen obviously wasn't.

"No, we're fine, thank you," she replied. I left them to it, went to boil another kettle, and came back to find Molly hyperventilating while Ellen was enthusiastically washing her "down below" (she actually wrote this in her log book).

"Shall I get Mother a cardigan?" I asked.

"No, she's OK," replied Ellen, continuing to flannel Molly's nether regions with vigour, and at the same time instructing her when to turn round, stand up and sit down. It was all too confusing. Molly needed time to work out what was required of her and even more time to decide whether she wanted to do it or not. By now, Ellen was ready to towel the rest of Molly dry, but Molly was heading for the doorway where I stood.

"No, don't do that to me," she whined. Ellen ignored her and kept rubbing. Molly gasped again and moved nearer the door. I took hold of her arm gently and said, "It's all right, let's just get this done, and we'll get you dressed and we can go out, OK?"

"No, I want to..." and she mumbled something unintelligible, but which I knew meant Get The Hell Out Of Here. All this time she was still stood in her bra and blouse, and stripy socks. She took a step forward. The next step, if Ellen or I resisted her, would be against me, and no way was I going to let the situation develop into a confrontation. Besides, this was my *mother* getting distressed, and my protective instincts came to the fore.

"It's all right, Ellen" I said, "I'll take her upstairs and dress her there." And I led Molly from the torture chamber, once her much loved bathroom, and we headed for the stairs. In the half minute that it took to move away from the hot water, soap and flannel department, a few more memory cells had died off, and by the time I had reached the bottom of the stairs I was able to persuade Molly to stand still while I put clean knickers on (her, not me); then her trousers. We went upstairs to choose a nice jumper, came back down to put on clean socks and sandals, and headed for breakfast in the caravan. By now she was fine.

Ellen left. I toasted and pilled Molly (finding out later that Wenna had already done both!), then left her in the van while I returned to the house to collect the dirty washing. As I walked upstairs, a little whiff floated under my nose. Oh dear. I recalled Sally saying You won't have to look for it, you just follow your nose. So I did. A small packet, non gift wrapped, sat in pride of place on the dressing table, and some dirty knickers were stuffed in an open drawer. I fled for rubber gloves and disinfectant spray, and the job (excuse pun) was done before I even had time to think about it.

(Those of a squeamish disposition can skip this paragraph ... but, in case you *were* thinking of it, and wondering, as John did, how Molly got a jobbie onto the dressing table without climbing up onto it, the answer is that she did it somewhere else, picked it up and relocated it).

Molly was by now as happy as a happy-house resident, and accompanied me to the car with a spring in her step. I drove her to Morwenna where the residents in the lounge greeted her with cries of delight.

"It's Molly!"

"Come on in, Molly, we're having a musical hour!"

"Would you like this chair?"

"Look at the little dog by the piano, Molly!"

"Would she like fish and chips for lunch?"

And Molly settled herself in the chair with a smile on her face while I checked out the toilet arrangements with the care assistant. All seemed in order, for the first time in my morning, and I was happy to leave my mother in the home's tender care.

* * * * *

Across the pond, holidays were high on the agenda too, but Jill and Adrian took their patient with them.

> *Just got back from Florida, and it really was a super couple of weeks. We could even leave Pob on her own for an hour or two, as she was quite happy to sit in the sun porch with her glass of sherry and watch the birds and lizards. She did put a damper on the proceedings at times, though. When we were at the condo Jacuzzi, she started to take her swimsuit off when she got out "because it was wet", so Jill had to frantically wrap a towel around her. As it happens, we had the whole place to ourselves but at least I was spared the horrible sight! The old girl is about a half century too late for antics like that in my book.*

> *One thing we sacrificed that week was the seven hours that we get each day while Pob is "at work", and a consolation of the holiday being over is that we get those seven hours back again.*

> *We are both ready for all this to be over, but still determined to stick it out. I fare a bit better than Jill, because as the condition worsens the old girl's world shrinks, and one by one people she knows get shut out of it.*

She ignores me more and more, and focuses on Jill, so it is much easier for me to hang onto my sanity.

Ah well, gotta go. Looking forward to that pint in Royce's pub. It has assumed the abstract proportions of the Holy Grail, a great golden foaming mug up in the sky, coaxing us ever forward towards freedom, happiness and normality.

Ah, if only a pint were all it took!

CHAPTER 22

BREAKFAST AT ... WELL, NOT TIFFANY'S, THAT'S FOR SURE

The care homes got us through the longest weekend, in spite of the problems, and Sally and I looked forward to more away-days for Molly on a weekly basis. We gave the staff at Morwenna a rough list of her likes and dislikes, telling them that she preferred finger food and fruit, and that she would do anything for cake, but I don't think anyone wrote these details down. At any rate, during one of the first weeks the staff reported that Molly didn't like her lunchtime chicken cobbler and had eaten only the pudding. This was predictable, but later she not only refused her teatime soup but threw it across the table.

Norma had told us a similar tale about Mavis and her trifle. Mavis, on a day trip to The Gables, was being slow with her lunchtime pudding, toying with her food, while everyone else had finished. The care assistant, no doubt frazzled, said, "Come along, Mavis, finish your trifle. You're the last one and I want the dish." So Mavis picked up the dish, grabbed a handful of trifle and threw it in the poor girl's face. Now, I am no expert, but if you were feeding someone who didn't finish their food, would you not just say, "Don't you want that?" and, if they didn't, take it away? I don't know. Maybe there was more to the story; all I can say is that nothing like that had happened at Parc Bush. Until the footbath episode.

Sally handed Molly her usual mug of tea one morning, and turned round half a minute later to find her pouring it over her feet.

Resisting the urge to panic, Sally kept admirably calm and merely asked, "Don't you want that?"

"No, I don't!" snapped Molly.

"Well, shall I take it?" suggested Sally mildly.

"*No!*"

There are times when mild will not do. Sally walked over to Molly and gave her fair warning. "I'm going to take it."

"No! I don't want you to do that!" For a moment it looked as though the tea would feature in a serious mug-of-war, but fortunately Molly gave in, albeit with very bad grace.

"Oh all right then, here you are," she muttered, and almost threw the mug at Sally.

So perhaps I am being too hard on the staff at The Gables, but at any rate, there is less of a health and safety risk throwing trifle around than in trying to give one's feet a hot flush.

We were not sure how far the Morwenna staff were actually trained in looking after dementia patients. On her very first visit, Molly had had an "accident" and had come home in not just clean clothes, but a nappy. Since she was not incontinent, and there should really have been no need for this, we wondered how often a patient was escorted to the bathroom, instead of just being asked 'Do you want to go?' Molly might not understand what was meant by the question, or might be in an awkward mood, or .... who knows? It was a problem we had to solve before she got to be the lucky winner of a longer holiday break.

* * * * *

The rest of the summer whizzed by, as it always does. Sally worked (or, as she said, went for a rest) several half days each week at the Crow's Nest and, on Wednesdays, all day. So, we arranged that I would come over each Wednesday morning and give Molly her wash and breakfast, while Sally got ready for work.

On the first Wednesday I got to Parc Bush early enough to find Molly still in the house, not yet having headed for the caravan breakfast bar. This was good news, as I was feeling valiant enough to wash her hair, and we were only yards from the bathroom.

"Coo-ee!" I cried as I opened the back door. Silence. I knew she was there, though, because I had seen her through the window.

"*Coo-ee!*" I bellowed, and reached the lounge where I found her engrossed in opening a large cardboard box. Ah! Her new mattress topper had arrived, made of that space-age stuff that costs £6,000,000 for lining a rocket but a mere £100 when thinly sliced and cut into bed-sized pieces. In view of the episode earlier this summer, when Molly's back had got her stuck in bed, we had decided that such a topper might be a good idea, being softer and perhaps easing the stiffness from which Molly suffered.

"Hi Molly," I greeted her. "What are you up to?"

"Just getting the tiffan tiddney," she replied.

"Oh good! This looks interesting. Shall we undo it?"

"All right," she agreed, so I got her to hold one end of the box while I tried to drag its contents out of the other. It was not an easy task, as the topper was rolled into a tight coil that clung tenaciously to the sides of the box, and Molly did not quite understand her role in the proceedings. The more I pulled, the more she kept walking towards me. At last the topper made its unwilling exit, and I was about to lead Molly upstairs when I caught sight of a dog shape in the sherb. Dear Charlie had come to see us.

I should just explain that Charlie was one of three new additions to the Ellis menagerie: a pair of Jack Russells acquired as hunting dogs for Martin, and a Dalmation puppy bought on impulse by Wenna and Toana. The Dalmation, Bernard, was a lovable mutt - that is, lovable to all but Martin who saw him as an unwelcome and not very useful tripehound - but he was sweet-natured, as were the

Jack Russells. Except that one of them, Jack, had a tendency to nip, and the other, this Charlie, was not house trained. There he was, crouched in poop mode among the hot house flowers, nonchalantly doing what all Parc Bush residents seemed to do.

I hustled him outside, and headed for the bathroom to fetch some toilet paper. A quick scoop, down the pan, and I turned to Molly once more.

She was gone. A glance through the kitchen window showed her retreating form heading at a rate of knots for the caravan where her breakfast awaited. Not yet, it didn't! I headed for the back door, and sent another erudite salutation her way.

"Yoo-hoo!" I cried, "come back here a minute! I need your help!" and was pleased to see her turn and come back, her curiosity piqued. I also saw Sally at the caravan window sniggering, the horrible woman.

Having put two kettles to boil (the immersion heater, as usual, being out of order), I got Molly to help me upstairs with the mattress topper, and together we stripped the bed, inserted the topper, and remade it. It all went quite smoothly, the only one to be disturbed being Bella cat who, having just finished her night's sleep, had snuggled down into the duvet for her daytime rest. She was not impressed by Tilly poking her nose in, and rewarded the dog's friendly sniff with a warning rumble and a heartfelt hiss. "Stop biddling!" Molly said to her, while I moved Bella's recumbent form onto a cushion in front of the window, and Bella settled down in a large patch of sunshine which was pouring itself in generous measure through the panes. There is a lot to be said for being a cat.

Now for the next hurdle. The hair. Last time it had been a real struggle, so this time I adopted a different tactic. I made no mention of haircut, wash, water, bathroom or soap. Instead, I poured a kettleful of hot water into the bathroom basin, mixed in cold, turned on the fan heater full blast and asked brightly, "Shall we do it in here?" The tone of my voice conveyed that she would know what I meant, which, of course, she didn't but I was pretty sure she wouldn't ask.

"Yes, all right." And in she trotted.

"It's nice and warm, isn't it?" The heater was by now melting the lino.

"Phew, yes! I think I'd better take this off." A bonus - Molly removed her coat all by herself.

"And we'd better take the jumper off too, shall we?" I added.

"All right."

"Now, you just put this on to keep you dry," and I put a towel round her shoulders, showing her how to hold it. She still had no clue what I was about to do.

"Now, just put your finger in there ... is that too hot?" The water was just warm.

"Oooh yes, that's much too hot!" .

"OK, let's put in some cold," and I made a great play of turning on the tap and doing lots of swirling, while keeping it more or less the same temperature. "How's that? That's better, isn't it?"

Without waiting for a reply, I ploughed on. "Now, just see if you can step over here ... that's right ... and bend down, like this ... keep your head over the water ... that's right! Great! Perfect! Now I am just going to pour a little bit of this warm stuff ... OK? ... Good. Lovely!" and with continuous positive noises and praise, I wet Molly's head, added shampoo, worked up the fastest lather ever, rinsed and, contrary to the bottle's instructions, made no attempt to repeat.

I gave Molly the towel and asked her to give her hair a good rub, which she did, more gently than last time. This was all going so swimmingly!

"Is that enough?" she asked.

"Let me feel ... just a little more," and Molly obligingly rubbed for another few seconds.

While I was on a winning streak, I brought in a chair to the warm room, sweat now dripping off me and condensation off the walls. Once she was sat down, I gave her the world's fastest hair cut, keeping up a constant flow of hairdressery inanities to keep her mind off the fact that she was being touched. Blow-drying took another two minutes, but Molly sat demure as a doll. Soon she was up, clean cardigan and coat back on, and headed once more for breakfast.

On our exit via the kitchen, we were just in time to note that Charlie had found his way back in and was finishing off Bella's biscuits on top of the chest freezer - where they were kept so that the dogs supposedly couldn't reach them. Charlie made his second exit that morning.

Molly and I reached the caravan, to be greeted by Sally in relaxed pre-work mode, Radio Cornwall going full belt in the kitchen, and Sally's friend Lorraine sitting on the far side of the room from nippy Jack, casting wary glances at him. Having greeted Lorraine, I walked towards the kitchen, but stopped mid-pace when I noticed my sister's jumper. It had a strange bulge in the middle. And the bulge was moving.

"What have you got there?" I asked.

"A baby ferret," she replied.

"Oh, of course. Silly me."

"Do you want to see it?" asked Sally, putting her hand gently up her jumper and producing one of Martin's socks. The sock was full, and wriggled. As Sally carefully peeled back the open end, a tiny, furry face was to be seen, eyes closed, whiskers twitching and miniscule nose wrinkling as it sniffed the strange smells around it.

"How sweet!" I cooed, whilst Molly peered over my shoulder to see what was going on. "Is it all right?"

"I'm not sure. It's the runt of the litter, and Mother isn't interested."

"Yes she is!" I replied. "Aren't you, Molly?" And Molly nodded her agreement.

"Not our mother, you idiot," said Sally, "the ferret's. Actually, now you mention it, I might let Molly look after it when I go out. She'll love it to bits." And with that, the sock was stuffed once more up the jumper, and I headed for the breakfast ingredients in the kitchen.

Molly's breakfast was quite simple, so, in between toasting and cutting the bread, dolloping on the butter, crushing pills and embellishing the canapés with copious amounts of marmalade, I had an interesting conversation with Lorraine.

"Why are you so wary of Jack?" I asked, as I stepped over a sleepy Clem in my path towards Molly. "I thought you liked dogs."

"I do," she replied, "but I got bitten by one just recently."

"Oh dear. Where was that?"

"On the bum," she replied.

"No, I mean, where were you?"

"Oh, it was at Cadgwith. I was minding my own business, walking across the beach and it just came up and took a chunk out of me."

"Jack wouldn't do that, would he Sally?" And I looked at the sweet little terrier sitting next to Tilly, both dogs eyeballing Molly as she crunched on her croutons.

"I don't think so," replied Sally vaguely, sorting through a pile of photographs on the table, "but he can nip if you put your face too near him, so I just told Lorraine to be careful."

Suddenly remembering that dogs should not be in the caravan at all because Molly feeds toast and pills to them, I persuaded a reluctant Tilly and Jack to join the guilty Charlie outside, then hastened to the other end of the caravan to shut the far door before they discovered that. Clem slept on while I continued stepping over him to feed Molly the remaining pieces of toast, followed by a bowl of melon slices.

There then followed a few minutes of complete silence - but only from me. Molly munched melon and chatted to the folk on breakfast television which was blaring from the opposite end of the room to Radio Cornwall, while Sally and Lorraine engaged in hysterical laughter as they viewed Sally's photos of a recent beach party. Their attention being thus engaged, they did not notice the visitor who must have sneaked in when I put the dogs out. Across the carpet, with slow, stately steps walked a chicken.

"Is that supposed to be in here?" I asked. One could never be quite sure in this place.

"Oh God!" said Sally. "No, it isn't," and she got up from the table and started towards the intruder. Her advance was initially impeded by Molly leaning down to offer the chicken a piece of melon, but she used this to her advantage. With one hand still nursing the sock-lump-ferret, she grabbed the chicken from behind as it considered the melon slice, and, with much clucking and squawking (from the hen), succeeded in tucking it under her arm. The poor bird froze into silence once it was clasped, and we no doubt added to her stress by stroking her ruffled feathers, but they were irresistible, so beautifully smooth and silky. Sally then carefully put the bird outside, where she scuttled off to join her sisters, no doubt eager to tell them of her narrow escape from being mugged and poisoned, and the dogs seized the opportunity to rush back in through the open door. As the next course was banana, which they did not like, they were allowed to stay. Still hopeful that Molly might produce something more to their liking, they sat with eyes boring into her, then their ears twitched as they heard heavy footsteps running up to the caravan, and they dived for cover as the door burst open and Wenna erupted into the room. The air turned a sudden shade of blue.

"For **** sake!" she exploded. "What is the ****ing matter with the man?"

"Wenna," warned Sally. "Do you mind? We have guests present. If you and your father have fallen out again, can you leave it till later?"

"I only said *one* word to him, and just because he's having to replace the ****ing thing ..."

"Wenna," I added. "Mind your language - please!"

"Yes, go away!" added Sally. "We'll talk about this later."

With one final expletive, Wenna was gone, storming off down the garden path, past Martin who was walking up it. He came into the van.

"What's she crying about?" he demanded. "I wasn't cross with *her!* I just broke the ****ing toilet seat as I was trying to fix it, and she ****ing storms off!"

"Would you like a piece?" asked Molly, offering some melon to the breakfast television presenter.

"I'm sorry, Lorraine," said Sally. "Martin, can this wait please?"

"Don't mind me," said Lorraine serenely, quite used to the tempestuous tempo of life chez Ellis.

"Sorry," said Martin and made his exit, still grumbling, while the air reverted to its normal colour.

"What was *that* all about?" I asked.

"Same as usual," said Sally. "Spotty dog Bernard."

"What's *he* got to do with a loo seat?"

"Nothing at all. Martin just gets wound up about him, and so he and Wenna are at loggerheads all the time. It doesn't take much to set either of them off."

Molly had sat calmly through all of this, and was now quietly sipping at a glass of cranberry juice, narrowly avoiding slopping it over herself when Charlie jumped onto the sofa and curled himself onto her lap. Lorraine decided it was time to go, said her goodbyes and cautiously edged out of the caravan past Jack who was now sitting staring into space, behind Tilly who was back on toast patrol at Molly's feet, and over Clem who continued to snore and wuffle his way through a rabbit dream.

The phone rang, and I got up to go, saying goodbye to my mother who sat serenely in the middle of all this chaos, possibly the sanest one there.

CHAPTER 23

HAVE YOU HEARD THE ONE ABOUT ...?

Sadly the baby ferret did not survive, in spite of being nursed very carefully by both Sally and Molly, and a miniscule grave was dug for it in the field, close to where Molly had buried dear old Bosun years ago. Molly forgot about the ferret immediately, and her attention was diverted, as ever, by Bella. One evening, Sally and the girls had been for a swift half jeroboam of wine down the pub, so popped their heads round the door when they returned, to see if Molly needed anything.

"Hi there," said Sally. "We've just got back from the pub. Do you want something to eat?"

"No, thanks, replied Molly, cuddling Bella to her. "We've just been there."

Bella would stay contentedly all day in the house on her own, since Molly would be ensconced in the caravan with a pack of dogs to keep her company. Dear old Clem, wheezing his way through his last days, little Jack and Charlie, Tilly when I visited, and Bernard the dotty Dalmation. On the day, back in the spring, when Wenna and Toana had succumbed to the charm of the puppy, they had agreed between them to share the care of their new baby, but what they had neglected to do was consult their parents. Although both girls were grown-up enough to make a decision, they were still effectively living *en famille*, and a few words with Sally and Martin would have been, to say the least, politic.

When confronted with this canine conspiracy, Sally and Martin's response was less than enthusiastic. They knew full well that the novelty would wear off for the girls and that they, Mum and Dad, would end up looking after yet another dog. They were also worried that a large, boisterous young mutt might easily knock Molly off her feet; since her summer cough and prolonged bed stay, she was quite tottery. In spite of the girls' protestations and promises, Sally and Martin did indeed often find themselves puppy sitting and poopy scooping, and for weeks Martin continued to fume and wave around threats of re-homing. Dalmatians are notoriously impossible to train, being several plums short of a pudding, and Bernard was forever in trouble. Sally, however, fell in love with the pup, even when he fulfilled all her expectations and grew into a dog yob, so Bernard stayed.

Molly, strangely, did not like him at all, and one day she and Sally espied him through the caravan window as he chased a chicken up the garden. Sally banged on the window, but it didn't stop him. "You should bell him around," said Molly malevolently. "Yes, if I get hold of him, I will!" agreed Sally. Molly also objected to Bernard pestering poor old Clem, whom she adored, and one day when the pup was being particularly obnoxious, Molly scolded him, "Go away, you burkey!" Wenna, just outside, heard this and burst out laughing, so Molly grabbed a newspaper, rolled it into a weapon and made smacking gestures with it. She and Wenna had a mock fight through the caravan window, and there was much giggling, but I actually think Molly was quite serious. We had learned long ago that confrontation was not a good thing, and could bring on violent reactions from an AD sufferer, and we were generally pretty careful to avoid any such thing. The newspaper fight was border-line.

Our non-confrontational tactics were borne out in another book I had just read, Learning to Speak Alzheimers. In view of some of Molly's vocabulary, I thought it might help us communicate in a general sense, although obviously not with direct translations, for that would be impossible. Who could make sense, for instance, of her telling Charlie, sitting cleaning his feet, "You won't be able to root your ennu when you go out."? Or of her asking Wenna, "Have you got my tubble steels there?" (Wenna replied that she would go and look for them.) But the book was more all-encompassing than mere communication, and I would recommend it to any AD carer. It promoted what the author called the habilitation approach, which I was happy to discover was what Sally and I had been doing for years, keeping the patient happy and minimising stress for any us. I learned other things too, not the least of which was that we were quite lucky with our Molly. She was not violent, awkward, or distressed, nor half as difficult as some AD patients were. So maybe we were doing something right. Or maybe she had not yet reached those stages. Whatever the reason, it gave us encouragement.

It was also interesting to see that the "further reading" section at the back of the book listed several autobiographies, written in the early stages of the authors' illness, just as Molly did with her diaries. Only she didn't know, when she wrote her diary, that she had Alzheimer's Disease. All she knew about were the black moods and depression when she was alone. How much happier she was these days! Even when asking Sally stupid questions ...

Molly to Sally: "Would you like some sick?"

Sally: "Pardon?"

Molly: (Giggle) "Would you like some sick?"

We never did find out what she meant, but it made her laugh anyway. And she had us in stitches when Royce and Patti made one of their welcome visits on an autumn afternoon. We were all sitting around the log burner in Martin's lounge, enjoying the warmth and companionship, when our nostrils were assailed by the most noxious emission imaginable from the bowels of Bernard. Royce, Patti and I, who were nearest to the hound, all pulled our jumpers over our noses, and as the smell wafted further up the room, others laughed and did likewise. Eventually it wafted as far as Molly. Patti nudged me and nodded in Molly's direction. She was sitting with her fingers stuck in her ears, but joining in with the general mirth, while the culprit snoozed on, oblivious to his crime.

Sally and I had the opportunity, briefly, to update Royce on Molly's misdeeds, most of which were just amusing stories, but he was horrified by our accounts of the summertime pony express.

"I just couldn't deal with that," he said. "You're a braver woman than I'd ever be, Sally!"

"Absolutely," I agreed. "It's all I can do to sort out the washing and clean clothes." I could see Royce was eager to change to another subject, but I ploughed on. "Yesterday I got Mother undressed, and she had no knickers under her trousers - and she reckoned her trousers didn't need changing!"

"Urgh," was all the reply my brother could make.

"I found the knickers in a little chest of drawers in the bathroom ..." I continued, and Royce smiled, "... plus a towel with suspicious brown marks on."

Royce reverted to another Urgh.

"It doesn't bother me any more," put in Sally. "I just scoop it all up and throw it in the washing machine."

"Yes," I finished. "Sales of bleach in Helston shops have recently sky-rocketed."

Although one might think that Molly's knickers took the starring role in the afternoon's conversation, the main topic was actually the wedding that was to take place in November. Patti's son Neil was marrying his lovely fiancée Jo, and the wedding reception would take place at Royce and Patti's Old Ferry Inn at Bodinnick. Since we would have travelled fifty miles or so, we were all invited to stay the night if we wanted.

When Royce and Patti first took over the inn, in December 1994, we had all turned up as a family to help them move in and string up the Christmas decorations, and in later years Molly spent quite a few Christmases there, washing up and helping out generally. This might seem a strange way to entertain one's mother at Christmas, but Molly was so much happier being a useful part of the team, that she greatly preferred this to just being an odd guest floating around, knowing few people and with nothing to do. It was only her bad back which stopped her seasonal slavery, as she could not stand at the sink for long enough to do a million dirty dishes. Then, of course, came AD, which put a stop to that, and lots of other things too.

So, for Neil and Jo's wedding, a placement would have to be found for Molly, and what better home than Morwenna at The Lizard? We booked her in for a total of five nights because John and I had decided to go on from the wedding to visit friends in Devon, while Sally and Martin stayed on at Bodinnick. Five days later, when Molly was collected from Morwenna, we learned that all had gone well until the last two nights when Molly had suddenly taken to wandering about the corridors and into other residents' rooms. Even this would not have been so bad, but in one of them she left her calling card. The rightful resident indignantly asked Molly to leave, and she wouldn't, so the care assistant was called. Molly had no trousers or knickers on, and her half dressed form was only removed with a great deal of gentle persuasion on the part of the assistant. So the naughtiest girl in the residential home was henceforth banned from spending further nights there. The staff could cope, but, unsurprisingly, the other ladies and gentlemen couldn't.

This incident put a stop to long term respite care for the moment, and perhaps, as I commented in an e-mail to Adrian, "This will finally put paid to your reveries of Molly, beaches and bikinis!"

Adrian did not comment on this, preferring to retain his dreams of long ago, but he had his own tale to tell of Pob's respite care.

A local paper has done an article on the day care centre that Pob attends. There are a couple of photographs featuring her, and the amazing thing is that she can read the article and still not have the foggiest idea what the place is or why she goes there. But she is still proud as hell that her picture is in the paper.

To add to her moment of glory, Pob, like Molly, had also been going walkabout, but her version was more successful.

I have always been pretty damn grateful for Pob's bad leg, because, although, sadly, it causes her pain, it prevents her from going for long walks. However, the other day, I was, with the companionship of a large bourbon, keeping an eye on her, when she announced that she was going to the shops, and that she was on her way to our house to get Jill. I told her Jill was busy but she said if that was so, then it was time for her to have a break. I was certain that Pob wasn't going to go through with whatever she had got into her head, because she can't remember a thing from one minute to the next, not to mention that she cannot walk more than a few feet without help.

I heard the front door open and shut. Right outside the door there are half a dozen steps which she normally needs help to negotiate, but she didn't come back in. A minute later, from where I was sitting by the window, I saw her at the mailbox pulling her mail out, so I thought that she would be back indoors in a moment. She wasn't, and when I got outside she really was heading off down the street to our house.

The incredible thing was that she was walking as strongly as she used to years ago. I followed her at a safe distance, called Jill on my mobile and she came out to meet Pob. The two houses are about a quarter of a mile apart, a helluva distance for anyone in Pob's condition, and our house is on a slight hill. It was this hill that did her in. She only just made it, with Jill's help, but even so, I would never have believed her capable of what she did. I was amazed that she even made it to the mail-box.

Given the same situation again, regardless of the very real risk, I would still not stop her. Poor old sod deserves a moment of glory, and she seemed so pleased with herself. Plus, for the duration of this event, about an hour, all her old personality, sense of humour and vim had returned.

This tale was amazing, but, as I understand from reading about AD, things like this can happen. Stopping short of anything quite so dramatic, Molly was nonetheless still capable of taking us by surprise. She was in the garden one morning, picking the washing off the line and folding it neatly into the washing basket when Sally came by.

"Oh my!" said Sally. "You are getting on well!"

"I'm not getting on," replied Molly. "Getting off, is more like it." This was exactly the sort of quip she used to make, so was her old sense of humour resurfacing for a moment? Or was her brain translating fact to speech as literally as it knew how? We could only guess.

Within seconds she was back into AD mode, commenting as she walked past the dovecote, "I suppose they've got a stonging plass somewhere." They might have, but who would know?

As she walked into the caravan, she caught sight of her reflection in the window, and started laughing. "Well!" she exclaimed. "I said about that and there's a piece over there, and it was me!"

All we could do was be glad, very glad, that she was happy and laughing, and rejoice with her.

* * * * *

Fortunately, respite care on a day-time only basis was still acceptable at Morwenna, and we continued to take Molly in for her Thursday treat of elevenses, lunch and afternoon tea. The visits were mostly successful, but she could get very irritable if left there too late in the day. When I went to collect her one evening, I could see from the lounge doorway her face of thunder as she sat on the sofa and glared at the television. This was understandable in a way - we all suffer from the dire programmes. But Molly was surrounded by old ladies who did not wish to indulge in conversation with her when they could not understand half of what she said. So Molly had no-one to talk to and nothing to do; she probably couldn't hear the television properly as it droned in the corner, and Sundowner Syndrome, the evening grumps, was well in force. She ignored me when I went in, and refused her coat when I offered it.

"No, don't fold that!" she snapped at me.

"OK," I said, and led her outside, where she shivered violently and said something unintelligible which I translated as, "It's cold."

"Yes, it is," I replied, "let's get this coat on and you'll feel much better." She complied, and we walked towards the car, but then she had trouble getting in, seeming not to know what to do with her feet. She managed it eventually, and then her mood lifted as she burbled away happily during the journey home and I replied as though I understood. When the local bus passed us at speed and I commented on how big and fast it was, she said, "Yes. It's about to go and out." "That's right," I replied, "but I suppose we'll just have to put up with it." She agreed again.

Once indoors, Molly went straight to the bathroom for a very long tinkle, which made me wonder once more if the staff at Morwenna were asking her often enough if she needed to go. I also knew that she had not eaten since lunch, as the young care assistant had told me "We don't usually give her tea, as she spreads it over the table," so I went over to the caravan to ensure that Sally had something for her to eat. She was already making up a plate of bread and butter and peaches, so I left her to it, as I had to get home to cook supper for John and myself. Having said goodbye to Sally, I walked off down the garden, intending to go straight to the car. But I had been spotted. Molly was watching me from the kitchen window, so I felt compelled to go in. Putting my head round the door I said, "Sally's just getting you some supper."

"Oh good!" she replied sunnily.

"She'll bring it to you in a mo. Don't you come out, it's cold out here. Just wait there and she'll be along in a jiffy."

"All right. Where are you going?"

"I've got to go home and get John's tea. I'll see you tomorrow."

"Oh good! All right."

"See you!"

And off I went, leaving her completely content and serene. Not a sign of Sundowner's. It was so easy to keep her happy. But it took time, and time we didn't always have. Neither, of course, did the care assistants.

* * * * *

In America, Jill's mother was further down Dementia Dale than Molly, so Jill and Adrian had been seeing The Rest Home loom large on the horizon for some time. So many emails contained the words, "I don't know how much more of this we can take..." that I expected any day to hear that Pob had taken up residence.

> The lapses are getting more frequent where she doesn't know who Jill and I are. I am "the manager", or her nephew or grandson, but, happily, not "my husband". This is a doubly narrow escape, because Pob is now reaching the stage where she is starting to hallucinate. Sometimes she will point out stuff that just isn't there, and while we used to think that it was a matter of her being unable to describe what she was seeing with the correct words, it now appears that she really is seeing something that only she can see.
>
> For a while, there didn't seem to be anything frightening or unpleasant in what she saw, but we really thought we had reached the end of the road last week. Pob collapsed in her bedroom and we had to drag her off the floor and get her into bed. Her blood pressure shot through the roof and she gasped that there was some kind of animal crawling out from between her legs and she had to keep on pushing it back. (Don't say it, Adrian, don't say a damn thing). Whether the hallucination was as scary to her as it was to us, I don't know, but she was fine next day and insisted on going to "work".

Apart from déjà vu experiences, Molly had suffered nothing like this, and we hoped she never would. But, by January of 2006, Jill and Adrian had taken a big step, prompted partly by a dream Jill had of her long dead father, in which he told his daughter, "*You are doing all you can, but there is going to come a time when you will have to put yourself first."* Neither Jill nor Adrian believed in messages through dreams, but they did believe in the sub-conscious coming up for air once in a while. On top of that, for all that Adrian and I had been sending relatively light-hearted emails for years, Jill's suffering had been more acute. Over the years that they had lived with Pob, Jill and Adrian had not left her on her own for more than a few minutes. They had no family to help, Pob would not accept a sitter, and from Friday evening to Monday morning, Pob would not let Jill out of her sight. Jill could not relax or read; Pob would be glued to her side wanting to help but not being able to follow instructions or communicate; conversation was virtually impossible, and the only respite Jill got was going back to a full-time, stressful job. On the basis of all that, I was not too surprised when Jill wrote the following to me:

> I have hoped, for the longest time, that I would be spared having to

put Mother into a nursing home, that she would just "go" in her sleep. And then one evening I looked at her sitting on the sofa, and I wished she were dead. The realisation of what I had just wished for appalled me. I told myself over and over that it was perfectly normal, but for days I kept reliving that moment, and hating myself for it. Then, once I got over the first wave of guilt, I started wishing she were dead several times a day, and these thoughts resulted in a depression the like of which I have never experienced. Fortunately, that seems to have passed, and now I'm back in the numbing resolve to see it through to the end, but I am so tired of feeling sad. This has gone on for such a long time, with no cause to believe there will be any improvement. Our lives are slipping by, and hardly being "lived" at the present time. My wonderful husband has always said that when it's all over, he wants to be able to look into my eyes and not see any guilt there. That way we can slip back into our own happy life. I pray it won't be too much longer.

It was obvious that some respite was necessary for Jill. This was a major development, because it meant that she and Adrian had overcome their mental block, shared by so many other carers - recognition that some step was going to have to be taken to alter the status quo. They made enquiries and luck was, for once, on their side. Adrian wrote:

> *It transpires that one of the women in charge of Pob during the day has a nice little sideline looking after Pobs over the weekends. What a blessing. This woman can give constant, trained supervision and, of course, Pob is already familiar with her. All the staff at the day care centre are so kind, and how the hell they do that every day for a living I am buggered if I know. They are all, in my humble opinion, angels. I feel that I have been in a lifeboat forever, and have just sighted land.*

And so arrangements were made for Pob to go and stay with her angel for a couple of days. Jill and Adrian could leave her with a clear conscience and no worries, and, as Adrian succinctly put it:

> *... we can disappear for our weekend ....HOORAY! ....YIPPEEEEEEEEEEE!!!*

Sally and I began to wonder if we should think anew about longer respite care for Molly.

CHAPTER 24

CLOUDS AND SILVER LININGS

As another year drew to its close, we had to think about making Christmas arrangements once again. The Ellis clan were going to be involved in a village event, with the local ladies cooking up a storm; John and I were happily resigned to our usual non-event, having had our party the week before when John's boys visited; Royce was out of the picture, as always; which left Molly's entertainment schedule. But it was no problem. We booked her into Morwenna for the three days of Christmas, and she had the time of her life. The Ellises delivered her each morning, she spent the day eating, chatting, enjoying the Christmas decorations and watching television, and I collected her each evening and took her home. The first evening I arrived at Morwenna to the evocative sound of a carolling choir, and I followed my ears to the lounge. There was Molly, sitting quite alone but cheerfully watching the choir from King's College on television, tapping her foot and humming along as they belted out Oh Come All Ye Faithful.

"Hello!" I greeted her. "How are ..."

"Shh!" she hissed at me. So I did as I was bid, and listened along with her. When the last *Chri-ist the Lord* had faded, she was happy to come home, and we did a festive tour of The Lizard village on the way, with its huge tree, Happy Christmas lights and electronically waving Santa. Molly loved every minute of it, even though Santa looked more as though he were shaking his fist at us. In times past, she would have noticed this too, and we would have shared a giggle.

The second evening when I arrived at Morwenna, Molly was in the dining room, busily engaged in putting spoonfuls of trifle into her cup of tea and stirring it around. The matron came over to remonstrate; a bad idea. She had told me only the night before that the staff were learning to leave Molly alone if she wouldn't co-operate; and now here she was trying to do something confrontational. I quickly saw that this would go nowhere, so I whispered, "I'll take over."

"Oh!" I said to Molly, as she plopped another dollop of trifle into the lumpy liquid. "That looks fun! Can I have a go?" and I picked up the cup and spoon before Molly had time to object. "Would you like to come and see the Christmas cake?" I added, putting the cup and spoon aside while Matron moved in for the trifle.

"Ooh yes," said Molly, ears ever alert at the word "cake". It was a beautiful confection, made with much love by the evidently talented staff. We duly admired it before we left for home again, Molly clutching her Christmas presents of a tin of biscuits and a chocolate Santa.

By the third evening, however, Molly had lost all her Christmas spirit. When I came to collect her, she was firmly ensconced in a bedroom along the corridor, shredding a paper hanky and refusing to come out. As she saw me, she momentarily ceased her shredding.

"Hello, there!" I cried gaily. "Would you like to come for a drive?" Of course she would, and she accompanied me in lamblike fashion, while everyone breathed sighs of relief. We did go for a drive, all round Lizard village again, to see the lights for the third night running, which to Molly was just another first.

The cold nights were bitter, and Molly had complained in like tone from day one, so every evening I took a sleeping bag with me and wrapped it around her shoulders as we walked to the car, and then over her knees once she was inside. She complained again, in spite of her wraps, as we walked through her front garden, but I distracted her by pointing out the pretty lights which Sally and the girls had arranged with creatively exuberant fervour. Electric icicles dangled right across the front of the house, strings of different coloured bulbs were draped high over the path and luminous flowery things bloomed by the front door. Molly smiled and nodded as I pointed, but became more animated at the sight of a banana skin lying on the ground. Someone had aimed at the compost bin and missed. "There's an armanu!" she exclaimed.

Soon Molly was in bed, with Bella, cake and a drink, and I switched on the television for her. We had thought about moving the television from the lounge, where Molly never watched it, to her bedroom some time back, but lack of an aerial had prevented our actually doing it. Then John suggested that we might not need an aerial, as the television had its own tiny one, and indeed this proved sufficient for channels 3 and 4. As long as there was a picture and some sound, Molly would be pretty happy, whatever was on. This became such a godsend that we were only sorry we had not done it sooner.

I must not forget to mention the Christmas presents. We gift wrapped all sorts of little bits and pieces for Molly, and she adored unwrapping them, taking ages and folding up each piece of giftwrap neatly as soon as she had undone the parcel. As well as knick-knacks and smellies, she had received some practical gifts too, such as some lovely, soft, woolly bedsocks. As she unfolded the paper carefully from around them, Molly examined the socks, held them aloft, and looked enquiringly at us. "What shall I do with these?" she asked. "They are for an old lady."

* * * * *

January was a fairly dry month, so Molly and I had quite a few walks, usually around Poltesco. I had to take it very slowly on the short drive down to the valley these days as Molly was uneasy with acceleration. It was not the actual speed, for she was fine at 50 mph or more, but the g-forces seemed to bother her. As we drove away from Parc Bush one afternoon, I had obviously overdone it.

"Ooh, I don't like it like this!" she exclaimed as the speedometer registered 15 mph.

"Am I going too fast for you?" I asked. "I'll slow down."

"Well, I don't want to macey you," she replied, "but I expect you'll find one."

As we turned the corner and drove past a line of telegraph poles, Molly observed, "Some of those have got bonks and some haven't."

"Mmm, I wonder why?" was my automatic reply while I considered what she might mean.

"Look, that one too!"

"Oh yes - and that one!" The penny dropped as I observed the telegraph poles more closely. Some poles had metal steps, for the engineers to climb, and some didn't. I guess that's what she meant. And I guess the engineers never knew they were up the pole, bonking.

As we walked along the Poltesco paths, Molly would jabber away all the time, sometimes using made-up words, sometimes words which were fine in themselves but which made no sense in reality.

"My mother asked if she would see me later, and I said I didn't know," she stated as we ambled along.

"Well," I answered matter-of-factly, "it depends how much time you have, doesn't it? You can't always do everything in one day that you'd like to."

"That's right, she said, then a little later added, "I wondered if I'd see my father, but ... (burble, burble) ... and I was singing - no, not singing ..."

"No," I said, laughing, "you wouldn't be singing, would you?"

"No! But if he was seen."

"Well, we'll wait 'till we get to the end of lane, and see what he thinks. Oh, look at that pretty little bird! Do you see him, up on that tree there? He's very noisy, isn't he?"

On another occasion, when Molly had been quiet for a few minutes, I dived into the family history myself, just to see what she would say, opening the conversation with, "Have you seen your mother lately?"

"No," replied Molly, which made perfect sense, as Nan had been pushing up the daisies for the last twelve years. Then, having thought about it, Molly added, "I saw her yesterday."

"Oh, and was she OK?"

"Yes, she was fine." She was going to tell me more, but something happened to distract us. Her next question came right out of the blue.

"Will there be a fanhawser when we get back?" she asked.

This stumped me so completely that I could only reply in the most general of terms. "I'm not sure; I suppose there might be ..." and then go on to another topic immediately. I never did find out what she meant, but Sally said she had heard her use the very same word. It is perhaps a credit to Sally's and my own neurons that we could remember the word; it was such a strange one that I was keen to include it in Molly's story, so I committed it to memory as soon as I heard it. I did this by picturing a fan and a large steel rope, as per the visualising method recommended by all memory experts. It won't cure AD, but it *is* very useful.

We walked on, chattering blithely, until a large tractor hove into view. "Here comes a damned woollid!" warned Molly, and we stepped into the ditch to let it chug past. We got back to our car a few minutes later and, as we had some time to spare, I gave Molly the chance to say what she wanted to do next.

"Would you like to go home now, or into Mullion to the shops?" I asked.

"I think the yammer," she answered.

Well, that would teach me! I now had a fifty percent chance of getting the next question right.

"You'd like to go shopping?" I hazarded.

"No ..."

"OK, you'd rather go home?"

"Yes."

Back at Parc Bush I asked Molly the usual question, "Do you want the toilet?" and she decided she did. I always left the bathroom door open a crack, just in case (although I was not quite sure of what), and after a minute I heard her say, "Oh, there's no green in here!" Peering through the crack, I asked, "No what? Oh, loo paper. I'll go upstairs and get some from the other bathroom."

"No, don't bother," she said. "I'll use this." And she picked up an empty toilet roll, used it, and lobbed it into the bath. Smiling to myself, I went off to don rubber gloves and find an antiseptic spray. Since she had only used the roll for number ones, it was no real problem, plus it was comforting to know that at least she did still wipe, and that she had the sense not to throw the roll down the pan.

We walked down the garden to the caravan, under a sky that now looked grey and threatening. "Is it going to strang?" asked Molly.

"It looks a bit like it, doesn't it?" I replied. "Let's get indoors quick! Where's the dog?"

"Charkey!" she called to Tilly who was sniffing at an interesting piece of chicken poo in the grass. Was I hearing things? Charkey had been our childhood dog, who had gone to his reward thirty-six years ago. Rather than actually asking Molly what she had said, I merely remarked, "I don't think she heard you. Try again."

"Charkey! Come here!" she called. The second calling was no more effective than the first, not just because Tilly wasn't Charkey, but also because she still found the chicken shit more appealing than us. However, what interested me more was Molly's word usage. It had been so many years since her long-term memory had followed her short-term one into near oblivion, I found it astounding that she could somehow dredge up a name from so long ago.

Sally found my Molly outings useful, not only because it left her free for an hour or so, but also because it tired Molly out a little - rather like Jill marching Pob round the shopping mall - so Molly was more inclined to sit still than wander about meddling, or tailing Sally. Hiding one's occasional irritation was not always easy, and it was often a relief when bedtime came, but Molly didn't always think so. When Sally suggested one evening that it was time to go back to the house, Molly accompanied her, but with an ill grace, grumbling and complaining that she hadn't even finished her drink of water. "Well, bring it with you," said Sally. Molly, grumbling some more, picked it up and followed Sally down the caravan steps. Just as they reached the bottom one, she had a better idea, reached out with the glass and tipped the entire contents over Sally's head.

After that, Sally kept a greater distance, or even passed bedtime duty to Martin, as he had invented a unique system. Standing just out of sight of Molly, he would knock loudly on the caravan door and say to an imaginary person, "Hello there! Oh, you wanted to see *Molly*. Yes, she's just inside. Molly! There's someone here wants to see you." Curiosity piqued, Molly would step outside, by which time she would have forgotten the "visitor" and Martin would say, "Shall we go over to the house, then, Molly? We'll fetch some tea and have a piece of cake." With Martin's method, getting Molly to bed was a piece of cake indeed.

We continued with the Thursday Morwenna run and Sally was thus able to do what she liked for the entire day. This happy arrangement had been in force for about six months when, as John and I walked Tilly down to Church Cove one Wednesday afternoon, we passed Morwenna and spotted a notice on the wall. It was a planning notification issued by the district council. The owners were about to convert the home into flats. I was puzzled.

"They must mean to convert *some* of the house into flats," I said to John. "Maybe for residents who are more self reliant than others."

"Well they're not wasting any time," he replied. "They've got the diggers in already." He was right; there was a huge machine in the front yard, that hadn't been there the last time I collected Molly, and beside it a pile of ripped up asphalt.

When I collected Molly the next day, I asked Matron what was going on. They weren't selling up, were they?

"Yes, I'm afraid so," she answered. "It's no longer a viable proposition. There's a letter on my desk for you."

I was too stunned to ask any questions. Besides, what could I say? We never did get the letter, and within a month the home was closed. Reactions were mixed; from resignation to panic to outrage. Poor Amie had the job of re-homing the permanent residents, who were not dementia sufferers and knew full well what was going on. There was not room for all of them locally, and some even ended up in St Ives, about an hour's drive away.

Running a care home is not the easiest job in the world, and there are two sides to every story, but this was a sorry little ending. For Molly it meant no more day respite care, since none of the other nearby homes were secure, i.e., locked doors to keep wandering AD patients within the grounds. However, as it was winter and Sally wasn't involved at the Crow's Nest, we didn't worry too much. We left it a month until the re-homing panic would have subsided, then phoned Amie. As always, the sweet girl was concerned for Molly and for us, and promised to make some enquiries.

Within days she had phoned again. "There are vacancies for day care at The Gables," she said.

"But that's in Redruth, isn't it?" I queried. It was where Mavis lived, and although Norma and Dudley had told us how good it was, it still meant an hour and a half to get there and back, twice in one day; three hours' driving for seven hours' respite. "It's not worth it, Amie." I said.

"Well," she suggested, "what about the one week's respite in six?" Although we had known of this system for some time, we had always preferred not to send Molly away for more than a few days, worried that she might be disorientated once she came home after a week elsewhere. Amie didn't think this would be a problem, however, and Sally was fully entitled to this regular respite which Social Services would (mostly) fund. So we followed up her suggestion, meeting first Clive from Social Services again, who filled out the requisite forms, then Ralph, a representative from The Gables itself.

Ralph came along to Parc Bush with an armful of yet more forms to be filled in, and to give Molly an assessment. Sally and I warmed to him at once. With many apologies, he asked us the same questions we had been asked a dozen times already, then proceeded to answer our own, setting our minds at rest on everything from breakfast to baths, menus to moods, conversation to confrontation. All the while, Molly was present, quite unperturbed by any of our conversation and even putting in the odd word or two if asked. Or even if not.

"You've got a lot of chocolates!" she said, looking out of the window.

"Have I?" murmured Sally, her mind only half on what Molly was saying.

"Yes, look" said Molly, pointing at the chickens in their run. "There are a lot of cubs in the dick!"

"Oh, yes," I said, looking out of the window with her. "Look at that one!" and we turned our attention back to Ralph. "How do you cope with gibberish conversation?" I asked him.

Ralph grinned. "We always respond. If one of our residents comes up to me, perhaps while I am working at my desk, and tells me all about something, in language that only he can understand, I reply 'Really? Did you do that? Goodness me' - stuff like that. They are trying to communicate with us, and no way should they be ignored."

Sally and I both nodded. "And how would you react to a seemingly awkward client?" I asked.

"Walk away," he replied promptly, "and try again later. If they are smashing up the happy home, leave them to it for a while. If they don't want to do something, we don't argue or try and make them. Our training tells us specifically; walk away."

"I suppose you have seen it all and done it all before," said Sally.

"I think so!" he smiled. "We have to be prepared for anything."

"What about the, er, unmentionable?" asked Sally, not quite liking to go into detail, but Ralph knew what she meant.

"No problem," he replied sunnily. "We expect the occasional little packet left for our attention, and we just deal with it."

The man was a saint. If the rest of the staff were the same, Molly was going to have a very happy holiday indeed at The Gables. With lighter hearts, we said goodbye to Ralph and, as he walked out, the dogs rushed back in. The newest recruit to the Ellis canine club, spaniel puppy Kia, jumped onto Molly's lap. Molly made a great fuss of her, and was so engrossed that she refused the cup of tea Sally proffered her.

"No!" she snapped. "I don't want that! I didn't ask for that!"

"OK," said Sally, calmly putting it aside. Turning to me she ground out, "I think I can feel an early night coming on for someone!"

Within seconds, the puppy had jumped off Molly's lap and found something more interesting to do. "Would you like a cup of tea, Mother?" I asked.

"Oh yes, please, that would be nice," answered Molly, and I handed her the cup that Sally had just put down. Turning to my sister I repeated, *"Yes, please, that would be nice!"*

Sally made a very rude gesture at me, but we both laughed. Molly was happy with her cuppa, Sally and I were happy with our mutual support, The Gables would be happy to give Molly her holiday. AD, at that moment, was not a problem.

CHAPTER 25

WHAT NOW?

I originally entitled this chapter "Quo Vadis?" (Where will you go?), but was told by my editor not to be élitist! I had used the Latin in honour of Molly's education and because, although her high school Latin lessons might not have been totally effective, she had always delighted in her "*Tacite, Puellae!*" to admonish us children if we were being noisy - and that included Royce, and the dogs of whatever gender. It had little effect in any case, but at least her education was not totally wasted.

In other directions, these days, of course it was. How could we help contrasting her excellent schooling, and continual eagerness to learn, with the vacant plot in her brain now, when we encountered the conversations I have written about in these pages?

I could continue for several more chapters with my tales of Molly, but where does one stop? There can be no sudden ending in this book, no dénouement to the story. Sally and I are well aware that no-one recovers from AD, that it gets worse, not better, and that one day we - Sally in particular - will find it all too much and will have to start thinking of putting Molly into permanent care. When we do, it will be the best care that we can find, and we shall continue to be thankful for her long, happy life, and to treat her remaining years with as much humour as we and she can muster.

In Pobland, Jill and Adrian were a step ahead of us, and the news I had been expecting for months arrived.

> *We have finally done it. We have stuck Pob in a home. Jill started looking just after Christmas, trying to find a place which wasn't a hellhole, and we recently got a surprise call from a place saying that they had a room vacant, and if we wanted it we had to move Pob in within 48 hours. It was a gift from the gods.*
>
> *We told the old girl that her doctor wanted her to go into a rehab centre to get some therapy for the pain in her legs. She agreed very readily, and I fully expect her to settle down nicely. But taking this step was traumatic. When we were taking Pob to the home Jill deserved an Oscar for the act she put on, but as soon as we were out of the room she bawled, and has since then cried so much that I think dehydration might become a problem. She swears that she will get over it, that her brain tells her it was the right thing to do, but her heart hasn't come around to that way of thinking just yet.*

Now it is Sunday morning and Jill has just returned from the home where she put in a quick visit to see how they treat Pob first thing in the morning. They are treating her pretty damn well, even taking her a cup of tea before she gets up "because she is an English lady". Everyone else gets coffee. And the old girl seems quite content to be there.

So far, so good. If she is really unhappy at the end of a month, we will bring her back home, but we both think that very unlikely. Meanwhile, an amazing thing has happened - I have barely touched the bourbon bottle. The lads at the liquor store are going to be wondering if I am OK.

Tonight, a couple of friends have invited us to dinner, and we can go without worrying about a "Pob sitter". That will be the first time in more than three years.

I sent an immediate reply.

"I think you and Jill are the bravest people I know. What a decision to have to make, albeit somewhat thrust upon you. I am not surprised Jill is going full flow on the waterworks, and am sure I would be the same, however much we have been treating the Molly situation with humour - some of it black. The whole situation is black, but I think it will very soon turn grey and then off-white for you both.

The main thing is that Pob should be happy and well-looked after. From what you say, she seems to be both. As for "giving up" the bourbon ... I give you two weeks at the most!

There's nothing else I can say right now, except that I too am sad, but mainly for you. It is the end of an era, and I am glad to have been a part of it, for mutual support and some smiles along the way. It's too soon yet, probably, but that pint is still waiting at the Old Ferry Inn."

Further emails from Adrian confirmed that Pob was indeed settling well into the nursing home, as happy there as she had been in her own home. The brutal truth was that Pob had not actually known where she was in either place, and Sally and I wondered if this would be the same for Molly.

The next email I had from Adrian confirmed that he and Jill had done the right thing.

Just got back from visiting Pob, and in the middle of a conversation which was mainly rubbish, the old girl looked around the room, and said "You know, this is ever such a nice room, I really love it here, everything is just how I want it." Wow!!!!

Much as I love my mother, I could not have done what Jill and Adrian did for so many years, or indeed what Sally still does, living in such close proximity to Molly. Besides people telling us that we were saints, one lovely lady even responded to my Molly Christmas letter by saying that we deserved a place in Heaven. That would be nice, but let me state here and now that we are far from being saints or angels. One's mother is a pretty important person in one's life, and it takes courage to break the bond, even temporarily, by taking advantage of respite care. But Molly is over 80 now, and she does not actually occupy first place in my list of priorities; John holds that. All the members of Molly's family have their lives to lead, and we must balance that with making her life as good as possible. I believe we have managed that, since Molly has now lived through twelve years of AD and is as happy a soul as you could wish to meet. How could we be sad or guilty about that?

As I was sitting at the caravan table recently, I was searching for something in my handbag and, when I eventually found it, I exclaimed, "Oh, here we are!"

Molly, chuckling, responded from her seat on the sofa, "Yes, we've been here since this morning."

I cannot help it; when she comes out with sparky comments like that, I find myself thinking that she is OK, all will be well, the improved diet is doing the trick, the pills are working ... she will return to the Molly we always knew: bright, witty, intelligent, inquisitive, caring, daring, fun-loving, observant, always ready to laugh. And yes, I know we remember the good points first, but we still remain very aware that she could be moody, irritable, puritanical, critical and hard to please, but heck, she is only human.

In reality I know, however many sparky moments remain, the slope we are on goes one way only. Downhill.

Why do I say "we" instead of "she"? Because we are there with her - our mother, our Molly, our pal - and we will stay together in this until the end. We don't know when this will be, how bad things will get, or whether we shall be able to keep her with us physically, in her own home, but we shall be there for her. We will keep her as comfortable, well fed, stress-free and happy as is humanly possible. And we shall make each other laugh. You bet we will! Because it's better than crying; because it's good for the health; and because that is how we have always coped in a crisis.

I hope you will be able to do the same, whatever your circumstances and problems. But in case you, or we, lapse, perhaps we should remember the following statistic that I came across on the Internet recently:

"There is more money being spent on breast implants and Viagra today than on Alzheimer's research. This means that, by 2040, there should be a large, elderly population with perky boobs and huge erections and absolutely no recollection of what to do with them".

Molly would love that.

FINIS

ADRIAN'S APPENDIX

1 May 2006
I have mentioned this before, but I am going to say it again.   It is about the restoring of the mother/daughter relationship.   Now, Jill is back to actually enjoying the old girl's company, because the personality has reappeared.   Not that the disease has reversed, of course that is not so, but putting Pob in that home has removed the dependency, fear, frustration, and all the rest of it, and I do wish that we had both known beforehand that this would happen.   The act of sticking the old girl in the home was truly rotten, and the pill would have been sweetened very considerably had we known the side benefits. So, because it might make the experience a bit more bearable for some other poor bugger ... **this absolutely must go into your book.**

OK, Adrian, here it is!